Got Sugar?

Complete Set of Three Books

Debbie Markham

Book 1

Got Sugar?

Philosophy of a Sweet Tooth

Comprehensive Lifestyle Guide
For All of Life's Delicious Journeys

Debbie Markham

Note

The information in this book is believed to be accurate and true at the time of printing. The author can not accept any legal responsibility of liability for any errors or omissions that may be made nor for any inaccuracies nor for any harm or injury that comes about from following ideas in this book.

© 2010 Debbie Markham

Comments welcomed:
debbie@functionablyhappy.com

To Nate and Zoe who inspire me

everyday.

And to everyone who has positively

influenced me in my constant quest

to turn obstacles into enriching

experiences, thank you.

Embarking on this journey of life is way

more fun sharing ideas, facing

challenges and brainstorming amusing

solutions with all of you!

Table of Contents

FORWARD

Many who have eaten my brownies, cereal treats, and other sweet delights have gone on to lead normal lives, enjoyably!

All joking aside, this book is not intended as medical advice. I'm neither a doctor nor a dietitian. For 25 years I've been soaking up health and fitness information like a sponge cake! There is so much written on diet, health, and exercise, and let me tell you, I've read it all.

It all began with a few file folders: one for recipes, another for diet and health, and the last for fitness and exercise plans. Before I knew it, I had accumulated a lot of sweet material. Through all this I learned that it is possible to maintain a healthy, strong physique while enjoying sweets daily! So, here, I want to share my lifestyle tips on doing it all, enjoying it all, having my cake, and eating it too.

The following is a collection of the best ideas from those file folders sprinkled with my own sweet philosophy on exercise, diet, stress, fun and life.

Bon Appetit!

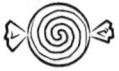

Introduction

"Sugar is the sun's energy stored in a tasty package."

My active lifestyle requires knowledge of what's best for my body. That said, I really enjoy life more with sugar. So I've decided to ride the line between healthy and unhealthy. Allowing myself to eat sugary things reminds me of my youth which makes me happy. I like to add elements of health to the desserts and baked goods I create; this way I still feel like a kid and can feel somewhat responsible too. For you, I want to be the voice of sugar-reason.

Many days I eat on the run—an apple fritter for breakfast, a granola bar for lunch, some pizza and beer for dinner. But that same week I'll do a 180—a fried mix of one egg and three egg whites breakfast, a salad for lunch, a dish of grilled fish and veggies for dinner.

Embracing my busy life, and accepting that I'll eat less nutritiously at times, knowing I'll flip back to my healthy ways, has made me mentally comfortable. In the back of my mind I'm always carving out time to be in the kitchen mixing, loving, and sharing delicious recipes.

Most diets fail because they neglect to address healthy ways of consuming sugar. I'm all about a lifestyle that supports balance. But remember, balance is a journey.

So there you have it, it's not an option for me to give up sugar. It's a matter of increasing components of health and exercise to balance out sugar consumption. It's about relaxing a bit, enjoying a perfect cake for all the individual components that are needed to create it. Thinking like this reminds me of all the sweet, rich, healthy, salty, dry, solid members of my family, and how each one, although unique, is needed to create our beautiful family tree.

I started compiling all this information in a book for myself once three messy file folders reached maximum capacity. Referencing them each week had become a nuisance rather than something I looked forward to when searching for ideas. Because it was rewarding to work towards accomplishing this task, completing this book, I dove in and never looked back.

As I told friends, they too were excited to see what I did to stay strong. It's hard to say if those closest to me were supporting me out of obligation or true interest, but either way, I thought, I'm going to write this for all the sweet tooths out there who are tired of reading the perfectly balanced daily menus that lack sugar!

As scared as I was to present my ideas, my genuine interest to just write what I know guided me. Over the years I've made lots of small, fun changes in my personal lifestyle. And I continue to look for silly ways to make me smile throughout my chore-filled, responsibility-packed days. Over time, I honed in on what things were doable on a regular basis, things that motivated me daily and helped me truly enjoy waking up each morning!

This book shares my habits (both healthy and indulgent), my mentality, and my observations which have really helped me squeeze all that great nectar out of life. I'm just an average girl who loves to eat good-tasting food as well as feel strong and healthy.

I encompass a love of all sports. I'm a curious reader of health and fitness trends. I frequent group exercise classes like yoga, Pilates, and pump it. I also practice solo-training (including training for triathlons and running races) and have qualified for the Boston Marathon. With insight from doctors and chiropractors, as well as physical and family therapists, I've gathered some great tips on keeping active and healthy. I'm also competitive—to the point where I find that making a game out of every workout, chore, or meal makes it more interesting! The underlying intent of my lifestyle is to have fun. And I do it while staying healthy and strong, and indulging my sweet tooth's desires.

While many nutritionists and trainers agree with various aspects of my healthy and sugar-filled lifestyle, some may not subscribe entirely to my interpretation of living the sweet life.

Experience it for yourself—see if you too squeeze all the sweetness of life, in every way possible!

Chapter One:

Cultivate a Healthy Mind

Acquire Knowledge

I enjoy the challenge of maintaining my weight in a world of increasingly delicious food and desserts. Knowledge fuels confidence, so I investigate vitamins, ingredients, calories and nutritional content of foods and watch what I eat. I also talk to people who know more than me and read anything (articles, brochures and books) relating to a lifestyle of health, strength, organization, and happiness.

There are many components to knowledge. Knowing oneself, knowing actual information, and also knowing how and when to use or share the information to inspire positive changes!

We all monitor our money daily, we constantly think of how we're going to spend it. We also plan how and when to save it, how to use it and where to donate it. It's the same with staying fit. Keeping track of what I eat reminds me of my bank account. I don't think of it as a chore or an annoyance, I think of it as being smart so I can enjoy indulgences without stress. This is a game I know works for me.

For example, by reading Starbucks' Nutrition by the Plate pamphlet as I wait in line, I know how to balance out my choices for the rest of the day, or how to order in the future when in a hurry. I was surprised and very excited to learn an apple fritter doughnut is similar in calories and fat to a zucchini muffin! This knowledge allows me to enjoy eating apple fritters, and helps me plan to eat veggies and protein for dinner!

Another example is realizing that one cup of Raisin Bran has approximately the same amount of calories and sugar as a Pop Tart or Take 5 candy bar. Cereal and Pop Tarts are fortified with vitamins, all three have the same protein and the cereal has the most fiber. But if I've eaten some whole grain bread and veggies for fiber, and taken my vitamin, I feel okay eating a Take 5 Bar or Pop Tart for dessert.

You can to gain more knowledge like this by reading online. Try to learn by reading online. A handy web site is http://nutrition.about.com/od/changeyourdiet/a/

calguide.htm. Type in height, weight, age and it shows your caloric needs. Another great way to learn is by using iPhone Apps. *Calorie Counter and Diet Tracker by MyFitnessPal* can help you stay aware of calories.

Research shows that people overestimate how many calories they burn during exercise. So, in order to avoid this miscalculation, I've learned how many calories different activities use and keep it in mind. I found some charts online stating the calories burned per exercise and duration. To find similar calorie-burning charts, type in 'exercise calorie calculator' into your favorite search engine. These charts are great because they take into consideration your weight. When I plugged in 200 lbs for 30 minutes of jogging, the internet chart said I burned 300 calories. When I input 130 lbs for 30 minutes of jogging, it said 200 calories were burned. Since treadmills don't consider weight, the calories they suggest being burned don't seem accurate.

I'm proud of my healthy eating habits. I feel I've accomplished something and then I'm excited to indulge in a treat because I earned it. I'm motivated to workout 30 more minutes for dessert. To me, it's like saving up—similar to not buying coffee for every weekday morning and getting a great new book each week instead. By working off those calories, I'm able to consume more calories in the delicious desserts that I love so much.

Skilled bakers, professional chefs, and chocolatiers are constantly creating irresistible pastries, hand-crafted truffles and delicious desserts! I love discovering new foods, especially sweet ones, so I'm always ready to fit in a workout in order to sample a new confection or innovative dessert.

Knowing myself and my propensity to go for everything new and delicious, I try to fit all my daily nutrients and vitamins in the smallest amount of healthy food I can. I aim to consume everything good that my body and mind need to get going, and still save room for the sweets I love! For more information on my savvy tips for integrating five food groups into meals and desserts, read *Got Sugar? Recipe Companion*.

To make a mental note of the healthy things you should be integrating into your diet, here's an updated, more accurate food pyramid. Keeping this in mind is just another game for me. I do my best to meet my body's healthy needs, but some days I need to carry-over my food choices to balance out other days later in the week!

Food Pyramid Guidelines

1 fat: This is a tough one. To keep it all balanced despite my sweets-intake, I keep active!

6-8 oz carbs: Sugary, bready, starchy, grainy things all fall under this category. For a benchmark amount, know that one slice of bread equals one ounce.

3 cups vegetables: So easy to integrate as a snack or into your meals.

2 cups fruits: Besides a great snack item, use them i breakfast recipes and desserts.

3 cups dairy: This usually equates to two glasses skim milk, one portion of yogurt or one portion of cheese.

5 oz protein: Focus on getting it through eggs, nuts and meat. If you're vegan, eating quinoa, sprouted seeds, soy foods or nuts with whole grains are also complete proteins. Think: one egg equals one ounce, two tablespoons of peanut butter equals one ounce, and a fist-sized portion of meat equals three ounces.

To my knowledge, it's best to eat a bit of protein with your carbs to minimize hormonal imbalance. To do this, try milk with cookies or eggs with toast, or simply exercise regularly. Blood sugar is in control when the two hormones (insulin and glucagon) in your blood are in balance. In response to eating carbohydrates, our pancreas produces **insulin**, the hormone responsible for storing fat or generating energy. On the other hand, both protein consumption and exercise produces **glucagon**, the hormone that promotes the activation and utilization of fat for energy. Check out glucagon on Britannica: http://www.britannica.com/EBchecked/topic/235785/glucagon, or other sources if interested in a more scientific explanation.

Also think about how you eat when you're not hungry. I do this occasionally, and I've wondered if it's some emotion propelling my decision to eat? Quite possibly if the desire to eat came when I was full, maybe I was happy, bored, frustrated or sad.

Since I run my business from home, food is readily available for instant comfort. When I get stuck writing, or become frustrated from a challenging photography portfolio, I've often headed for the bag of chocolate chips. I don't feel guilt, I just make a mental note about needing to exercise for two, not just one, reasons: to maintain my strength and health, and also to use up that extra fuel.

I might feel guilt when I get home at 9pm from a dinner out with friends and I realize how much I overate and drank socially from feeling happy. I still have to practice eating less of the gigantic portions that are served in most restaurants. But ladies, it's all a work in progress. We've got to eliminate the guilt and just move forward with finding a solution.

One way I do that is by knowing it takes a 3,500 reduction in calories to lose 1 pound. For me this equates to eliminating about 500 calories per day for 7 days. I like to split the amount and reduce my food intake by 250 calories for 6 days, and add 30 more minutes of workout for the other 250 calorie use, in order to avoid just eating 500 calories less per day.

I hate getting to this point, we all do. But when I get there, I move past the guilt and the problem, and commit to a healthy streak for a week. I write down food I've eaten on a notepad that I can leave for myself on the counter as a reminder. This helps me stay aware of the calories.

Keeping a food log definitely helps you realize your calorie intake. You might not realize how much you snack on your kids' foods! I know I didn't until I starting keeping a log. All of this comes back to the importance of knowledge. Be aware of how much and what you are eating. Be aware of slight weight gain, before it might get out of control. Know how to keep a food journal to constantly stay aware of your health and diet. Know how to keep that protein-and-carbs balance, in order to feel happy and avoid feeling lethargic.

Also, by staying aware of my food intake, it's like a game and my mind stays active: calculating, analyzing, and assessing my history and future strategies. This is essential so that I don't get too caught up in the results. Don't fret and sweat the big stuff, make a plan, use your brain, work toward that goal, and before you know it you'll be on your way in no time.

Yes, I wonder if I'll be able to meet my ideal end goal, but distracting myself from that large, looming goal ahead, which can be really daunting, with small attainable little goals is a great solution. I play little games with myself in order to reach those small goals and it helps me move along with an upbeat manor through each week.

With each small goal I've achieved, I feel rewarded. By letting go of that end goal, I don't let myself get down and frustrated if I don't lose the 3 pounds I was aiming to lose. *Just as important* as achieving the end goal is enjoying the attempts with small goals and games. Try to recognize all your mini-successes, so that whatever the outcome you'll feel positive and balanced. Know that you really did try your best and you won't get discouraged, annoyed or frustrated with trying it again.

Trigger Notes

After gaining some new knowledge, I may want to adopt a new strategy or system. To remind myself of this newfound discovery and plan, I tape reminder notes to my refrigerator and bathroom mirror. Taping reminders or trigger notes around are a great way to make sure your brain practices thinking in a new fashion. This way you're prompting your brain to form the habit or pattern that you want to develop.

Reading things once or absorbing knowledge once isn't enough to make a change. Continually reading and practicing healthy habits is how I make my healthy-shift stick. I read up on affirmations and learned they really do help. They really do promote positive change and positive mental attitude.

Notes that I've made in the past range from improving self-motivation and self-worth to simply remembering new habits. Here are a few that I've taped up, which have made a positive impact:

- Thoughts aren't real. Stress comes from believing in unnecessarily worrying thoughts.
- I am the perfect body for me.
- Make up a new game while doing a chore.
- Trust the phenomenon of life.
- Laugh at my brain—I don't ask it to create thoughts.
- Accept compliments. Give compliments.
- Life is filled with delightful surprises.
- Hug my kids four times a day.
- Believe in myself.
- I am lovable. I love.
- Stop eating the kids' leftover breakfast.

Basically, we all have behavior patterns that we use automatically to respond and react to our lives. Humans wouldn't have survived if we didn't learn what worked and what didn't. Since we need to be able to respond quickly to the environment and events around us, our brain references the past to make quick decisions. These are our learned responses and thought patterns. If some core behaviors, from which other responses are built, were formed in a situation not needed for today's survival, the "still" brain keeps referencing them. This makes it difficult to evolve into the mentally healthy direction that we aim for. By choosing to think optimistically and say positive affirmations, we will subconsciously refuse those outdated core behaviors and begin to reassess them. For me, affirmations worked! My mind realigned its thought processes by thinking about the statements more often, until they became an integral part of my lifestyle.

On the flip side, there's just so much to know! And health advice seems to change almost with every new generation of scientists. If I really think about it, scientists have their own set of behaviors and beliefs which color their research and results. So, in effect, the advice we cull is often subjective—you can't say that one piece of advice is the ultimate fact or the ultimate truth.

Almost as a contradiction to what I've tried to encourage you to think in terms of the importance of acquiring knowledge, I learned that it's just as important to give up knowledge. Be ready to reassess your thinking, your thoughts, that facts you thought you knew. After all there's always room for inight, as with everything in life.

By understanding and accepting that you'll never know the ultimate truths and mysteries about life, you'll be less confused. And by enjoying constant learning and editing that knowledge base, you'll be able to enjoy maintaining your fitness, health, and positive attitude. It's all part of the process. I feel better day-to-day armed with knowledge, as well as the understanding that it's very subjective and needs a grain of salt. In the end, I trust my intuition after all the knowledge I've accumulated.

Debunking Sugar Myths

Sugar has received a bad reputation over the years. But think: all carbohydrates including starches and sugars originating from foods like bread, peas, corn, pasta, fruit, candy bars are technically sugar, not just what's in your sugar bowl. Now, can all those things really be that bad? Let's reformulate our thoughts about sugar to get a more comprehensive understanding of what it is.

When consuming any carbohydrate, the digestive system breaks it down into simple sugars (glucose), which are carried through the bloodstream to nourish and energize cells. Whether or not it was from eating table sugar or a carrot, by the time it gets to the liver, it has been broken down to a glucose molecule. There's no way your body knows that the glucose molecule came from a carrot versus a grain of table sugar, except that the entire body benefits from more nutrients when consuming the carrot.

I've been scared by claims about how horrible sugar is to our bodies, so I began to research sugar online. The information is sometimes baffling and contradictory. Here are some thoughts on a few of the most intriguing, hot debates on sugar.

Myth: Sugar causes hyperactivity in children

I don't want to be the outcast mom, or be known as thoughtless when people see me allowing my kids to eat something sweet. So, I found many different studies from universities and clinics that concluded that there is little evidence that refined sugar plays a role in hyperactivity for most children.

1. Does Sugar Make Children Hyper?, by Robert Needleman, MD, FAAP, http://www.drspock.com/article/0,1510,4126,00.html.

2. Another study published in the *New England Journal of Medicine* (http://topics.abcnews.go.com/topic/New-England-Journal-of-Medicine)gave some kids sugared foods and others foods with artificial sweeteners. No notable difference was found.

3. Questions posed to the specialists at *Cornell Center for Materials Research* offered some more answers: http://

There seems to be no sugar rush. So why does it appear that kids get hyperactive when they eat too much candy? The affect is more likely from the caffeine. Caffeine is found in chocolate and some sodas and increases any person's energy.

Myth: Sugar causes cavities

I was really baffled by this, so I'm glad that I learned what's actually going on! Sugar can lead to tooth decay, so brush well and often. Floss, drink water or chew gum regularly after sweet treats, and cavities will less likely form.

But did you know sugar itself doesn't damage teeth? Several types of bacteria are present in the mouth that feed on sugar. When bacteria metabolizes sugar, it creates acids in the mouth which de-mineralize tooth enamel leading to decay.

Sugar at normal mealtimes does almost no harm to teeth because the exposure to sugar is not sustained and the other foods you eat tend to scrub your teeth clean of sugar. Fresh fruit is rarely a problem, even though it contains natural sugars, due to the cleansing effect of the fruit fibers.

Myth: Sugar consumption displaces other nutrients

Sugar is a relevant ingredient in many healthy foods. Several U.S. diet surveys showed that the consumption of sugar has little impact on vitamin and mineral intakes.

Vitamin and mineral consumptions are determined by the whole diet, not a single ingredient like sugar. That's why it is important to eat a variety of nutrient-rich foods. If people ate only corn, their diets would be deficient in most essential nutrients.

Myth: Sugar makes you fat

Sugar has only 15 calories per teaspoon and is no more fattening than any other 15 calories. Weight is gained by taking in more calories than your body burns for energy. Carbohydrates (like sugar, bread, fruit, and potatoes) and protein provide 4 calories per gram. Fats provide 9 calories per gram. One problem with sugars, however, is that many products add a high amount of sugar to sweeten the products. This, in turn, causes the product to be higher in calories. Because consuming more calories means you must expend more calories to reduce or manage your weight, this can be of concern.

Myth: Sugar causes diabetes

If you have diabetes, you do need to watch your sugar and carbohydrate intake to properly manage your blood sugar level. However, if you don't have diabetes, sugar intake won't cause you to develop the disease. The two main risk factors for Type 2 diabetes are being overweight and living an inactive lifestyle. Eating sweets does not cause diabetes. Inactive sugar lovers, however, may increase their chances of obesity, if more calories are consumed than burned each day. Inactivity and obesity are associated with people developing Type 2 diabetes.

Positive Habits

I've definitely aspired to integrate many positive habits, like practicing self-acceptance and demonstrating unconditional love and patience with my kids. But who am I kidding!

I can't actively and simultaneously maintain all the ideal positive traits and healthy habits that I dream of having. I have to admit, when I do succeed at maintaining a healthy diet, daily workouts and professional goals, I feel rushes of adrenaline, pride, and self-worth, which as you know feels incredible. But I can't keep that up year in and year out. So in order to continue being positive even though not hitting super-woman status on a weekly, daily, hourly basis, I need some more manageable expectations that I'm a allowed to meet, and I need some time off on ditching the food pyramid.

It's my constant goal to be aware of and monitor my moods, actions, and reactions to see when I feel best, though I may not perfect them daily. Food awareness as well as goal setting and game playing are fairly regular positive habits that I maintain for myself. And to keep myself balanced and happy, there is one positive habit that I stick to without fail: my daily exercise habit.

Everyone needs a primary positive habit as well as other positive habits that you're keeping up fairly regularly. You can't be super perfect as you may plan, but you can set goals and do your best to achieve them.

For me, daily exercise is the number one, primary positive habit that I maintain in order to feel great. Without the routine of daily exercise, I feel less happy. Endorphins don't flood my system and I lose momentum. I feel healthier, if I'm strong. As a result of my commitment to my positive habit, my confidence is boosted too. This then fuels a positive cycle. When I'm confident, I feel proud of myself, I'm positive throughout my day and I'm a better mom.

I haven't always been this habitual about exercise. After college, I wasn't biking to class every day and bopping around campus. I noticed I felt kind of melancholy and weak after a day of work in an office. In order to stop this state of being, I needed a change. So I decided to establish a new pattern of activity.

Almost 20 years ago, I started jogging and biking daily and started logging my feelings. I logged the exercise and hours in my day planner and assessed my state of being at the end of each week. Since then, I've trained myself that I must exercise for mental and physical well being, no matter what! It's a positive lifestyle habit. This habit has helped me eliminate wasting time and brain space on deciding whether to work out or not

—I just do. No thought needed, no questions asked. I simply wake up and I know I'm going to exercise (unless it's my one day off that week) and I know that I'll reap the benefits of a happy heart, positive mind, and healthy body (unless it's my one day off that week.)

Like most women, I've been through a lot in my life— getting a divorce, having best friends move away, losing relatives and dealing with job changes, not to mention changing hormones while needing to maintain composure through serious adult responsibilities. All these instances, that could present a lot of stress in life, needed to be balanced out with some positivity. This cemented even more the importance of exercise for me.

No matter how I ate, which job I had or didn't have, how poorly I reacted to my kids temper tantrums, or how I dealt with the newest crisis, I knew I would exercise and this would help me feel better. Knowing that I have one positive habit, knowing that I plan to achieve something, knowing that I'll do something good for myself no matter the troubles I face—this has surely saved me.

So, aside from needing exercise to balance out being highly interested in sugary things, it has helped me keep my confidence. I have stayed strong physically even when personal disasters have mentally paralyzed me.

Enjoy Everyday Life

Positive habits can help our perspective on life be one of enjoyment instead of annoyance. Beyond having a primary positive habit that grounds you in moving forward, other ones can be imbued throughout your daily life. For instance: try making chores a positive experience. Something simple like grocery shopping gives me joy.

I find product placement intriguing. I used to work in marketing so I love thinking about product designs, logos and where items are placed on the shelves. Some pay to be placed on prime shelves, some don't. I can relate to those smaller companies, since I'm also a small fish in the pond in terms of my own business and profession. So, out of empathy, curiosity, and if not solidarity, I support those small guys by buying products from their off-beat brands. Small habits like this make me happy and reinforce positivity.

I also stay positive by being organized at home. To stay organized, I keep a list of kitchen staples that I need to keep mealtimes going for my family. Each week I'll note the kitchen staples missing in my fridge or cupboards, and I'll use this once a week for a few meals (see 'Kitchen Staples' in *Got Sugar? Recipe Companion*). This means I'll spend less time on grocery shopping. Less time grocery shopping means I'll get more free time to fit in a workout. This is another game I play—I set a limited shopping time as a goal, and when I achieve it, I'm rewarded with more free moments. Another great aspect of this way of shopping is that with a steady flow of set choices, I get to engage more of my creativity. Say you only have cans of beans, tuna, black olives, and artichokes. Not sure what you could make out of it? I'll say, 'There's my sandwich!' I'll just mix it up with olive oil and put it on some whole grain bread.

You might wonder why this cognitive re-structuring and habit building doesn't work for diminishing my sweet tooth. It can. But I just love eating sweets—they make me feel giddy. I love savoring all the flavors and emotions that come with eating sweets. I simply enjoy making a game out of organizing my time to create them and equally enjoy staying active in order to earn them.

I appreciate all the artisan bakers, pastry chefs, chocolatiers and candy makers out there. I also love to bake. Creating a dessert brings happiness to my friends and family who enjoy the ritual of my offering! I won't lie, it makes me feel good to see others enjoying what I've made. I don't want to give up the joy I feel when creating or consuming a perfect balance of sweetness and texture. For me, this pleasure transcends so many different levels and aspects of my life that I've just taken it on as a part of my life. And really my healthy attitude is not mutually exclusive. I've made them work together and dovetail nicely so that one simply complements the other.

If I want to eat two delicious pastries for breakfast, an ice cream shake for lunch and have wine with dinner, I can do just that! Ok, I'll have gotten little if any nutrients, calcium or fiber. So to make this day nutritionally balanced, I'll drink 9 glasses of water throughout the day, take all my vitamins, and eat three prunes for fiber. I'll feel great having got all my nutrition, and happy to have enjoyed such luxurious treats as well. This would make me all the more motivated to do a great workout the next day!

Most days I enjoy trying to burn sugar off! I play a game, like an arcade game in my mind—and try to use up the calories I've put in. If I have to exercise 30 more minutes to use up that 300 calorie brownie sundae I ate, then so be it. I wake up 30 minutes

earlier and zap it out as energy expended,
remembering how I enjoyed my decision to eat it.

Big-Picture Goals

In order to do it all—gain and adopt new knowledge,
create positive habits, and make the most out of daily
life—you should create some big picture goals. My
main picture goals are:

1. Schedule time for daily exercise.
2. Be mindful of diet and calorie intake to
   maximize enjoyment of sweets.
3. Keep creating and learning lifestyle tricks, and
   playing games to increase metabolism, pride
   and self amusement.

Exercise Induces Positivity

Studies have shown that exercise brings about
significant increases in confidence and self-esteem.
Both aerobic exercise and resistance exercise suppress
appetite hormones and postpones hunger for about
two hours. Whenever I don't exercise, I'm hungrier and
more likely to fall victim to snacking. I'm here to
reassure you that you can stay fit and consume sugar

within reason. Doing it both is definitely feasible. Don't feel guilty, simply embrace it: be happy and do both!

Now, we know that exercise releases the hormone glucagon which helps offset insulin levels, which in turn helps you avoid an energy crash and stay physically pumped. Also, I find that exercise helps me cope and combat mental exhaustion. Mental exhaustion and physical exhaustion are two different things for me. When I am mentally beat, I find that doing 10 minutes of yoga, my night time circuit or walking the dogs really revives my energy level (read '15-minute Night Circuit' on page 37 for more). But don't take my word for it, try it out yourself! Physical exertion seems to actually help my mental fatigue!

Many times I'm mentally exhausted from meeting client deadlines, staying up late as I edit photos until 2 am, and sleeping less. Getting up at 6 am to walk the dogs and then working out before my kids rise for their school day at 7 am is challenging to say the least. But, every time I dare myself to resist the urge to snooze, I'm rewarded with pride. On top that, it gets easier each year!

Having a plan for exercise really does make all the difference for me! Here's how I stay on top of my exercise schedule:

- **Plan my week of exercise.** Each Sunday evening, I take 10 minutes to plan the following week. If exact times are written on the calendar, I don't back out. It's no longer about whether or not I'll do it. I will get the exercise in because it's planned. Even though I have a flexible schedule being a photographer, I also volunteer, coach, and write during the day. So in order to get my exercise into my busy daily schedule, I usually exercise first thing in the morning.

- **Keep the calendar visible.** I used to have it on the kitchen counter, but then my counter became cluttered. So, I bought a giant 24 inch x 36 inch entire year plastic calendar. I use a dry erase pen, can see the big picture of my year and absolutely love it. I map out short and long term plans (and write down the date of the event I'll do, as my training goal.)

- **Exercise with a friend.** Often I find that exercising with a friend can be entertaining: whether it's keeping each other company as we take bathroom breaks or joking about the exercise video we're doing. I was a solo runner and biker for years and being accountable to someone else is a great motivator. The soccer and softball teams that I coach hold me responsible for keeping active and fit. My healthy schedule is important to others—I feel needed, and feeling needed really feels great!

When I first started running with another marathoner, I learned that exercise buddies are invaluable for turning sessions of grueling training into fond memories. She was as beautiful a girl as any I'd ever befriended-sporting gorgeous teeth, skin, nails, makeup and hair. She wore pearls and beautiful clothing and kept her home and car immaculate. Within a month of running two to three times a week we were hacking, spitting, snorting, and farmer-johning side by side. The second month as the runs got longer, we were even relieving ourselves in random places. The silly times we shared definitely made those training sessions more enjoyable, especially because I didn't think of her as a hacker, spitter or road-side reliever!

- **Exercise early.** Although the thought of running at 6 am in the dark used to scare me, I have been rewarded a thousand fold with all the gorgeous sunrises, misty, ethereal landscapes and traffic-free routes. I've enjoyed the reward so much that I now actually prefer to exercise early. It gets it out of the way, so I don't have to schedule it in or think about it later. I occasionally swim with a masters swim team from 5:30 am to 6:30 am. It's awesome to see the sunrise around me as I turn to breathe, and being around other active men and women ages 21-60 is great energy to start off the day! It raises metabolism and I gotta say, I do feel peppier all day. British research found that cyclists could hold a harder pace for longer at 6:45 in the morning than at 6:45 at night. You have a store of energy that you can fully utilize before its get tapped into by all your other daily activities. Besides being more energized in the morning, the exercise will give you more strength and motivation for the rest of the day.

- **Find a happy place.** Since music inspires me immensely, I enjoy downloading it and making new playlists each month. When it comes time for my workout, I look forward to putting my earbuds in and taking off into another reality!

- **Pat yourself on the back.** Keeping a mental journal works for my motivation. But a good friend of mine takes note of her successfully completed workouts on a calendar with little symbols that work for her. She'll note '3R' for when a completed 3-mile run, or 'L' for a completed session of lifting. At the end of the week we're eager to reflect on our accomplishments by reviewing our physical efforts all week long, especially if we've indulged over the weekend!

Keep Reading

Aside from reading fitness and health magazines when I'm in the bathroom (that's where I stack them up), I read each night to inspire myself as well as relax. Even if it's just a single page, I'll get some reading in. There are three books on my nightstand at all times; two books relating to personal growth and one fiction.

For 15 years, I've been an avid reader of self-help, inspirational books. In my late 20s I went through a period where I was overworked at a corporate job, then moved away from all my family and friends to open my own business in a new town, which was stressful. But by jumping into life opportunities, I got to know myself.

Through these difficult life changes, I learned techniques to feel accepting and loving of my abilities to make choices, and to lighten up in order to enjoy what I used to think of as stress. By reading great advice, I learned to create a peaceful inner state of being, one which brings me fulfillment that's completely independent of my external environment— whether it's calm or torrential, I'm centered, balanced and peaceful. This has been a continuous and integral part of my life.

Beyond reading about mental, emotional and inner well-being, I read about physical well-being. By reading up on physiology, I'm on track to stay healthy and active. It's during quiet reading times that I'm reminded that counting calories and portions are just games my mind plays. I don't need to get too serious about record keeping. Just have fun being aware of all aspects of health (including nutritional content and calories) and be aware of how the mind can interpret those things. Sometimes, the mind gets carried away with information, and might start obsessing over a single detail, fact, or goal. That's not healthy so let it go, stay aware and keep moving forward. Usually I laugh at what bubbles up in my mind, realize it's the mind's job to solve problems (imaginary or real) and continue to read inspirational books to further develop my happy, healthy mind.

There is so much interesting information just waiting to be harvested and taken on board. It feels great to continually educate and improve myself with this information! But after awhile of reading philosophy and personal growth books, I need to dive into fiction.

Reading fiction, on the other hand, is equally important. Fiction sweeps me into another reality, pulling me away from my daily duties, plans, thoughts, and worries. In this way it calms me. Fiction also exposes me to a new experience, a new way of seeing something, a new place, a new culture. This fresh, different take on life, helps keep me on my toes so that I integrate new positive ways of looking at the world and my life.

Realize Positive Intent

Life is like a great movie. All people are characters in it and they are probably doing what they think is the best decision. I know I'm doing what I believe is positive for myself and the world. Sure, I feel mad, disappointed or annoyed sometimes when things don't align exactly as planned. But I try to laugh at my reactions and smile at how passionate my feelings can be. I breathe in my aggravated feelings and acknowledge them. Then I let them go by immediately baking, reading a page in an inspirational book, cranking out 15 push ups or doing something in which I know I can excel. When I dissipate the negative feelings faster, I can get back to feeling proud and confident, which makes me even more determined to keep practicing my positive habits!

I jump in and open the door to whatever positive direction life is unveiling. I try my hardest, fight for what I believe in, and don't give up, but I've consciously developed a habit of letting go of whatever outcome. Sometimes life throws you hardships and sometimes you don't achieve your goal, but you've done your best and this is what counts.

I give my all to practicing positive habits and working towards maintaining a fun, active, encouraging, balanced, happy lifestyle. That's all anyone can do, right? I've spent 10 years practicing this concept of believing—that with a small seed you can develop positive intent.

Life offers so many possibilities and it's no fun to be stalled by the fear of the result being sub-par or not what you expected. By believing that whatever result *is the right one*, I'm able to leap into more adventures and enter more discussions because I believe every action leads to the right outcome. In this way, I'm constantly trying and learning new things. This gives me an open mind, and with an open mind, I am less judgmental since I've seen many ways work for the better.

I'm reminded of a Chinese story called "Good Luck, Bad Luck!" where things that seem like bad luck (their horse runs away) turn out to be good luck (when it returns with a herd of horses.) And how good luck (new wild horses) turns out to be unfavorable (the son breaks his leg trying to tame one) which leads to good luck (the son not being drafted when the army comes for abled-bodied youth.) My take away: don't try to judge anything. If I catch myself placing a "good/bad" label on things, I recognize it now, because for months I taped up the phrase "no good, no bad" on my bathroom mirror. By thinking this way, you can let go of feelings (easier) from your mate not noticing your needs, hearing people talk behind your back, not achieving a goal you set or not making that traffic signal because your mind takes it less personally. *Who knows* if it's good or bad luck - just keep acting with positive intent and believing that the outcomes are destined to be whatever they are based on your intent and other influences in life, and that's all you can do.

Healthy Sweet Tooth

A sugar-injected healthy diet is satisfying! I drink milk with my cookies. I add chopped spinach and walnuts to brownies. I make sweet treats with healthy items like fortified cereal. Knowing I'm getting something of nutritional value in my sweets makes me feel great.

Pulling together daily family dinners aren't always easy as pie. But I grew up enjoying the family meals we ate together at the table, so I want to keep this positive tradition going. For the most part I try to ride the line between fun and firm. I catch myself saying things like 'Get your elbows off the table' and 'Sit up straight, don't lay down next to your plate.' I also find myself wishing it was time for dessert.

After all, dessert puts everyone in a good mood. It always amazes me how well my kids behave when dessert is at stake. This is just one more reason to eat it every night!

At the dinner table with my kids, I try to ask a question or have a contest relating to health and sweets: 'Whoever finishes all their veggies first gets five chocolate chips', 'Does cake have any nutrition in it?', or 'Where does sugar come from?'

If I don't know the answer, the kids and I do some research. We'll look things up online or discuss the possible answers during our meal. These kinds of games at meal time are so successful because they engage the entire family. By the time we have dessert, we're functionably happy, having fun.

As a mother, just as in other arenas in life, I want to be playful and amusing as well as serious and knowledgeable. One without the other makes like too mundane.

> *"I learned that courage was not the absence of fear, but the triumph over it."*
> -Nelson Mandela

Challenge Fears

We're all creatures, living here on earth, afraid of a variety of things relating to our personal history. But the more times I face a fear and get past feeling anxious, the more I feel liberated. I'm having way more fun feeling uncomfortable and later elated by my attempts, than I was just settling for where I was and feeling regret and wonder.

Recognizing that I'll either feel fear (if I'm going to attempt something new or challenging) or regret, (if I choose not to engage in the opportunity) has led me to take on challenges more and feel the effects of fear. I prefer feeling uncomfortable from overcoming a fear, than feeling uncomfortable from regret or wondering if "I should have". This way I get to learn a lot of new things along the way of overcoming a fear, which expands my knowledge base of things possible on earth. Expanding knowledge leads to increased understanding and acceptance of the variety of ways people choose to live!

I have two school-aged kids and no employer. Managing my own business, I challenge fears and battle self-doubt daily. I must keep working hard and pursue my passions of photography and writing to earn this lifestyle I so enjoy.

I think the power of positive habits is kicking in here, since I'm writing the *Got Sugar?* series. I've thought of dozens of reasons why my books aren't needed in the world, that they're not unique enough, that the information's already out there. But since I'm practicing challenging my fears, I've kept at the mission, and here are the fruits of my work.

Same goes for exercise: Whether I'm taking a new class at the gym or attempting a faster pace than I think I can do, I just try it. I might try it for a short period of time and give myself an out-option if necessary—but at least I still go for it. Many times I'll just hang in there and end up surprising myself by doing better than I thought I would. If it turns out I'm less embarrassed than I thought I'd be, I feel proud in tackling something outside of my comfort zone.

When I started college, I had no waterskiing experience. A boyfriend taught me how to get up on one ski on our first spring break. Soon after, I joined the waterski team at University California of Santa Barbara. Seeing 18-20 year olds excel at waterskiing techniques and tricks was truly eye-opening! I leapt into a new, exciting world, a world of waterskiing, sport, and challenges. Discovering these sportswomen and sportsmen, discovering the sport, and discovering all that I could learn from waterskiing was truly amazing. I'd never known this community and these events even existed, until I gave it a try. Quickly I learned about ideal body-form for slalom courses, skiing tricks, and ramp-jumping. The more I was exposed to, the more I soaked up every experience. I learned how to master the different speeds of the boat for any event at waterski tournaments and practiced everything I was taught. I found it so rewarding to improve a skill. By my senior year, I knew how to drive a ski boat at various speeds and I competed against other colleges. This sport was one of the best parts of my college experience. By taking that first step and trying something new, I bonded and grew with 20 fun, smart, hard-working, water-loving people.

Fast forward to this year when I visited Park City, Utah for a reunion with my college roommates. Throughout the course of my college career, I had gained seven wonderful roommates. And now we get together annually for a long reunion weekend. We went to Olympic Park to watch the freestyle aerial skiers train for their jumps off long ramps into a huge swimming pool. This is how they practice with the lack of snow during the summer.

When entering a local museum on one our play-days, I spotted a sign that offered three-hour classes to the public. My heart skipped a beat as I excitedly decided to join. I signed up before I could talk myself out of paying $95. In no time, I was practicing jumps on the trampoline into the pool. Then with ski boots, skis, and a helmet on, the instructor pointed up the stairs I had to climb with the simple words, 'go for it!'

Standing at the top of the ramp, I thought, 'This is going to propel me straight up into the air.' This was something new, the jump was quite high. The thought of it was exhilarating and unbelievably scary all at once. I knew I just wanted to do it. So I let go, trusting the physics of the ramp and keeping my eyes level with the horizon. I flew down that ramp and jumped! The feeling of being airborne was like no other feeling.

By the end of three hours, I had accumulated a number of unsuccessful jumps and some really sore quads. But all in all, the experience was amazing and I had accomplished all three of my goals: complete a 360° helicopter move, a back flip, and a front flip.

Had I not joined the waterski team back in college, I wouldn't have launched off that wood ramp in Park City. Every person I've ever met, every book I've read, every experience I've participated in, every time I actively listen, I'm rewarded for challenging my fears, whether immediately or later in life. Each attempt opens doors that wouldn't have opened.

Beyond physical activities, stepping outside your comfort zone in your relationships at work or at home is also important. Discussing money issues with roommates, talking about hurt feelings between family members, or confronting parents or coaches regarding fairness in sports can definitely stretch limits and prompt awkwardness. When addressing whatever problem at hand, I try hard to view myself as a character in a movie, and wonder how the awkwardness will turn out. After all, these little bumps keep me interested in life.

So with any difficult challenge, whether physical, work related or emotional, the best motto truly is Nike's: just do it.

> *"Leap and the net will appear."*
> -A Zen saying

Don't Worry, Be Curious!

There are probably hundreds of ways to diet and lots of different books and articles on strict no-sugar diets, fasting diets, no-dairy diets and cookie diets. You name it, it's all been written.

Since I like to keep myself amused and entertained with life's routine activities, I've tried many styles of dieting and working out. I don't worry. I'll just try it because it's different and because I'm curious.

I am intrigued by the creativity behind these different diets! Don't beat yourself up with worries if the new diet you want to dabble in doesn't work out. Obtaining knowledge through a variety of sources and trusting feelings of well-being is all a person can do. Experimenting will help figure out what feels the best!

For awhile I tried the no-carb diet. I ate as little as two slices of turkey for breakfast, tuna on a bed of lettuce for lunch and normal dinner. I felt remarkably full for how little I'd eaten. Several weeks passed and then I realized, 'I liked my life with sweets, I'm not this rigid.' I like baking and feeling like a kitchen scientist! I know myself better and have chosen to compensate in other ways to stay strong and healthy to make my life work for me.

Get Sugar!

Sugar comes in a variety of forms. Yes, in the edible form, but also in the form of love! I receive sugar from my friends and family and am endlessly smitten and utterly grateful. I give and get sugar from my kids with their loving hugs and their desire to play with me! In my home, we like to say, 'Gimme some sugar!' or 'Who wants some sugar?' as we spread the love! Finding ways to give and receive sugar in the form of love makes life sweeter yet. And I find that sugar always results in me getting some sugar in return!

When my son hit the end of 2nd grade, he stopped responding to my over-zealous good-bye hugs and professions of love for him at drop-off. I felt the you're-embarrassing-me vibe. So, we made up a game so he doesn't have to say 'I love you' in public. We agreed that when I drop him off curbside at his grammar school we would look into each other's eyes, hold it for 1 second and smile big as we say yelled, 'Byyyyyyyyye!' As long as I have something that equates to an 'I love you, mom!', I'm good!

Another thing I'm increasingly aware of is how fast time goes by. If I don't plan a daily tradition with my kids, before I know it the day's gone and I've gotten no sugar-loving! All of a sudden it's time to make dinner, sit together for a meal, shower, read, and shove off to bed. Having seen many days end up like this, I started a ritual of making something together as soon as they got home from school. It ranges from peanut butter balls to pumpkin bread for my son, and from angel food cake to chocolate chip cookies for my daughter. Regardless of the result, we work together for 10-15 minutes creating something. After that I work in my office, as they complete homework assignments. As a reward for our dedicated effort we have a freshly made treat that we'll reconvene to consume!

I keep adding positive habits one at a time, as they relate to a need I have. The tradition above evolved because I needed to share more sugar, or love, with my kids. I needed more bonding time that didn't have a reason. We have to do homework, we have to go to practice, we have to do chores, etc. I wanted to create time together where we weren't just pulled together for some task. So, I sat and thought what I could do with both of them, in a short amount of time, which would create a lasting memory and give me a short-term love-fix. Cracking, mixing, melting, kneading, rolling, cutting in the kitchen works for me. For one of my college roommates and her kids, a board game or drawing time works. There's no right answer. There's just continual change as kids grow and my life develops. We just need to review the change and adapt to meet these new needs. Everything shapes me. That's why it's important to review the small things in life. These are small ways I can make myself happier while being responsible. If I'm not doing things to bring me joy through my chore-laden days, it's not shaping me or my family in the direction of more joy when the next changes happen.

I'm excited to see how I'll change my daily habits or traditions to fit my family's needs next year, then the next, and the next. I look forward to the challenge of adjusting to change and the heaps of sugar that will come.

Chapter Two:

Lifestyle Tips and Tricks

Fly like a hummingbird, darting lightly through each day, looking to experience the core sweetness of all people, places, things and situations of life.

Life gets mundane. Life gets busy. Life is serious. I'm a single mom and a professional photographer. My daily life requires a lot of planning, responsibility, and a great big heaping of level-headedness. Accomplishing my dreams—well, most of them—as an entrepreneur and a mother is what keeps me sane!

From the big things like volunteering at the grammar school or coaching my kids' sports teams, to the things that often go unnoticed like finding the best health insurance rates for my family or making sure my kids have clean underwear. With school functions, work, sports and the duties incorporated into home-life, my calendar is like a jigsaw puzzle.

While facing the responsibilities of adulthood can be draining, life can be entertaining when you embrace a child-like spirit.

As discussed before, one of the ways I stay upbeat is by practicing playfulness while accomplishing my goals. I set challenges and play games that remind me to sip the nectar in whatever situation. It's easy to get sucked through a blur of life by the fast-paced world.

To keep life light and keep myself entertained, I'll bring out my child-like spirit when doing the simplest things. When withdrawing money at an ATM, I'll distort my lips in funny ways for the camera. It's also great to think that I'm the only mom who does such crazy things to stay child-like. I need to laugh, or I find I'll start resenting my adulthood, wishing I didn't have to grow up to be in charge of so many things. Anyway, a simple thing like making funny faces makes banking much less of a chore, I'm a right?

I even get a kick out of my self-induced competitions that inspire me to move faster and make the most of my tight schedule. Some mini-competitions include clocking my dishwasher unloading time, and trying to beat the time each week. 'I am such a geek,' I think to myself often. Interestingly enough, the more often I embody the geek in me, the happier I am completing my tasks. The more meaningless games I come up with, the more fun games bubble up in my head without even trying, as I journey through life. And I get the added benefit of laughing at myself when I come up with some of the ridiculous games that I usually do.

I also think, 'Why not?!' I'll just try some new made-up game to see if it can be done. I also think, 'I wonder if anyone else has ever unloaded the dishwasher this fast, or on their tippy-toes, or with one eye-closed the whole time.' The whole process is silly and fun and that's the point. Injecting some of this light-hearted spirit is what keeps me balanced in the sea of routine, chores, and responsibility. When you make things silly and fun, it's no longer just a duty.

Just doing something amusing amuses me. When I do something creative, fun, silly, daring, joyous or uninhibited, I'm living in this moment. I'm focusing on having fun in the present, no matter if I have duties and chores. I'm having fun now, I'm laughing now, not later, not postponing it endlessly, not ever smiling and having a laugh because I never get around to it. This is what game playing is about for me—living for the now.

The more I do it, the more it happens naturally, and it becomes a positive habit.

My job affords me the flexibility to engage in these random lifestyle games I talk about in this chapter; after a photography shoot I can wait and edit photos after my kids' bedtime and do it until 2 am if I need to.

If you work 9-5, you won't be doing your work with one eye closed or nipping away to get your swim workout in during afternoon public lap times. But many of my habits can be incorporated to some extent, however infrequent. Try them out at home, make yourself laugh at your desk, share a silly moment with your coworkers.

Time-savers

The main thing I need is more time. I need more time to do all the things I have to do, all the things I'm curious to try, all the things that I want to do as a loving parent. So first thing's first, find time to do everything, and then you can find your way of incorporating the fun.

Here are some things that I do to free up time for baking, my family tradition, and exercising, my main positive habit:

- **Buy ice cube trays**: Use these as jewelry organizers. Two will stack on top of each other in the drawer. Annoying, time-wasting searches for earring pairs has become a thing of the past!
- **Learn computer commands**: Every time I open or close a window, or copy and paste text, I look at the shortcut commands next to its name in the pull-down menu. Now, I do Command+C for Macs or Ctrl+C for PCs, in order to copy (and countless other commands)instead of dragging my cursor up to the menu bar and clicking around. This saves me precious minutes.
- **Shop on-line:** I do this occasionally to save time. Instead of driving, parking and getting sidetracked by cool sale items, shopping online is direct and quick. I keep a notepad by my phone and wait to gather a group of items for one order. Many web sites offer free shipping over $50. I shop at local stores to support them as much as possible too.
- **Play games to move faster**: I time myself when grabbing a jacket for my kids who are

already buckled in and then suddenly realize they forgot to grab it for school. I time myself when unloading the dishwasher or washing machine. The kids have fun timing me, making me sprint. I lunge and dart around to beat the last time. I do this with a smile and my kids think I'm fun. I get the chores done faster and have more free time to exercise. I'm telling you it's a win-win situation.

- **Exercise two days a week at home**: For me, this saves me 20 minutes driving time R/T.
- **Brush my teeth in a different area of my house each day**: This one's pretty creative! While brushing with my right hand, I walk around and organize stuff with my left hand. I'll tidy all my medicine in a cabinet, I'll throw out expired stuff. As I'm brushing I'll tackle the kids' bathroom, I'll change the dirty washcloths, throw out the old toothpaste, and wipe off their counter. Super time-saver!
- **Use canned beans and frozen veggies**: For everything from soups and chilis to main meals and side dishes, these will save you from loads of prep time. No need for washing and cutting, simply plop them in and you're ready to go.
- **Type a list of birthdays and important events, and buy cards in advance:** While waiting at a car wash or other random time-

zapping errands, I'll grab these cards so that I don't have to go out to buy them at the last minute in the future. It feels great to be organized, and when it comes time for someone's birthday, I'm thrilled and proud of how prepared I was!

- **Eat energy bars for lunch.** When traveling or errand running, I always pack an energy bar: I substitute it for lunch. Doing so gives me more time for sightseeing and walking around or errand-running since I won't have to sit and wait at a restaurant! And since other cities and countries have unusual, unique desserts, I always want to save some room for trying these out. By eating an energy bar for one of my meals, I'll have more room for dessert!

- **Group errands or chores:** When I drive out of my small town to the nearest Mac Superstore, I plan to swim laps during the window of available public times, hit Costco, buy any known family birthday present needed in the next month, and grab pet supplies. Bi-weekly I need crickets for my tree frogs' diet. I've been known to strategize my errand runs so well, that I don't ever backtrack as I loop around town. If the pet store is open, earliest, I'll hit them first, then Costco, which opens next. Then I take my ventilated plastic carrying case full of

30 crickets into the pool locker room, since the car is too hot in the sun. They'll chirp and sing for an hour for showering and changing women —how cute is that!

Perfecting Music Playlists

Musicians are my heroes. Their ingenuity of beats and lyrics continually inspire me. Since I like doing things to the beat of music, I make different playlists for each type of workout. After years and years of working-out daily, I need a constantly updated variety of music to stay fired up.

In order to find out what song will work best for a certain type of activity you need to figure out a song's BPM (beats per minute). To figure out a song's BPM, count the beats in 10 seconds of the song and multiply it by 6. If you count 20 beats in 10 seconds, then multiply 20 beats by 6 to get 120 BPM.

Weights Playlist

Test out your lifting pace to see what beat you enjoy most. Take biceps for example: I lift up for two beats and down for two beats. This works out to 120 BPM, so

I would choose a song with that BPM like Phil Collins' *Sussudio*.

Aerobic Activity Playlists

Steady or Mellow Pace
Feel the beat of a song for a more relaxed aerobic workout. When your foot hits the ground, or pedal goes around, find a song to match your pace. For me, 80-82 BPM matches my pace for steady runs or cycling. Nickelback's *Someday* is a good example of a song with 80 BPM.

Speedier Pace
Interval training (an intense burst of speed followed by an easy pace) is an important aspect of muscle conditioning. Having songs to match that faster pace makes it more enjoyable; it helps me focus on trying to stay with the beat. Lily Allen's *Smile* is a good one with 96 BPM.

Push-It Pace
Once you know the BPM that you comfortably run at, let's just say 70 BPM, go find three songs at that mellow pace. Then find another three at a pace slightly higher, like 75-80 BPM. Arrange them in an alternating pattern, so that you get a push-it song after your

mellow song. This way, every other song pushes you to run a tad faster than your normal pace.

To keep up with a faster beat, make your steps shorter; don't take big strides, little shuffles are good, just hit the beat. If you'd like to test a push-it pace, try Black Eyed Peas *Pump It* which has 77 BPM. Even if you don't like the song, you'll be able to hear the beat easily.

Being in the car with the radio turned on is tons more fun when trying to distinguish a song's BPM. While driving, I listen and count out the BPM of new songs to go home and download.

> *"The quickest way to become an old is to stop learning new tricks."*
> -John Rooney

Everything's a Game!

Creating positive habits, for no other reason than to entertain, induces more interesting results! Life is an adventure, professionally and personally, and I try to recognize and jump into the adventure every day!

When I started playing games to amuse myself, I never would have guessed it would have evolved into such a mini-goal-oriented-daily-fun habit. But I found that the more challenges or goals I created, no matter how incidental, the more feelings of pride surfaced. If I won or succeeded, I would be happy and not bogged down with all the responsibilities bestowed upon us with adulthood. In order to achieve many of my goals professionally, I've had to reach out and ask for help. This scares me, so I stand up whenever I make nerve-racking phone calls to new or distant friends when networking and searching for advice. Standing up and pacing a certain spot in my house sounds silly, but knowing it's my game, gives me comfort. Now the game has changed to see if I can stop pacing within 3 minutes, down from 5 minutes earlier this year.

Exercising for 30 minutes a day in itself is a great game. But taking it easy the other 23 hours and 30 minutes doesn't give me energy or strength and it doesn't help me burn off the sweets that I love. So, I began to view every activity or chore as a game. By doing 30 seconds here, a minute there, it helps make my life way more entertaining; I amuse myself and my kids. Because I act like a kid daily through these games, I also feel less annoyed about being an accountable adult weighed down with chores and responsibilities.

Another thing I think about when consciously choosing to run around, is how Native Americans must have lived, always active, hunting, and gathering. Life was more physical in the past, and for people today our lives are centered on a lot of sitting in offices. I sit a lot for work, I sit while writing, I sit while editing photos. This is not active. So I make sure I exercise through playing these games. I have a lot of fun trying to simulate the life of an active hunter or gatherer in my little games.

Yosemite always reminds me of what life must have been like before the turn of the century. I can't imagine being an early settler in the winter. They must have had to keep moving just to stay warm! Hiking with my kids, I found myself curiously watching the time it took us to hike half a mile uphill at a normal pace. Then we figured out the half-way mark on the map and guessed our arrival time, selected a lunch break spot, and estimated the total time for our 7-mile hike.

This may seem like no big deal, but having the big picture in mind kept morale boosted. These goals, though inadvertent, gave us something to talk about as we hiked. We stopped many times to enjoy the views, gather sticks, and dip our toes in the river's edge. We guessed several times how long various lengths of our journey would take. How long would it take to get up to that ridge? Could we make up for lost time if we'd spent time gazing at waterfalls? Besides witnessing the obvious beauty of Yosemite Valley, we felt elated by our accomplishment. The light-hearted spirit and our mini-goals helped make the 6-hour uphill playful and enjoyable.

Active Games

- **Digging holes**, boogie boarding and collecting shells and sticks. I do whatever my kids do at the beach. The trick is to keep up with the kids' pace!
- **Sliding** with socks on my hardwood floors as I run between rooms. Remember, *Footloose*?! Yeah, you do! Let that inner rock-star in you free!
- **Trotting with the shopping cart and hopping onto the foot bar** as you go from the farther end of the parking lot to the store entrance. It's entertaining to see other shoppers have a double take as an adult glides by on a shopping cart.

- **Focusing on foot speed**. Trot upstairs using every step. Next time trot up stairs skipping a step. Time which one was faster. When my kids are loaded in the car off to school and yell, 'Mom, I forgot a jacket,' I can bound upstairs without wondering how much time I need. I know because I timed myself already! Oh, yes! I feel awesome when I get that jacket in as little time as humanly possible. And in the near future I'll be timing them! But currently, since they're not seasoned fast-jacket-retrieval sprinters, I'll play the game myself.
- **Playing hide and seek.** Tip-toe silently and slowly for 10 minutes as the finder. This engages leg and core muscles as you do so. Surprising the kids when you find them is good clean fun!

Chore-related Games

- **Washing dishes on my tippy-toes** without falling. After 10 minutes of it, spinning and lunging occasionally for interest, your calves will feel it and your heart rate will be elevated!
- **Unloading dishes or laundry using only one arm** for one minute. Then only the other arm for a minute.

- **Loading the dishwasher one item at a time** really fast to engage my abs. Grab each item from the sink, turning fast with a tight core to load the machine, then reach back to the sink, and repeat. This means that I leave dishes in the sink for the whole day, just so I can play this game with as many items available for a full two minutes for maximum abdominal action!
- **Folding two baskets of laundry before the next commercial break** or timing myself as I fold a load of laundry. I can try to beat it next time.
- **Bicep-curling with grocery bags** as I carry loads into the house. Or I just might see if I can carry all the bags in one trip to test the superhero strength of my upper body!
- **Picking up the pace** when raking leaves, doing light housework or gardening. Grab tools quicker, move faster and have fun trying to do chores faster than normal.
- **Making organization a game.** I challenge myself and my kids to find the most matching socks in the laundry pile, or to set the table in under a minute. We'll try to add different goals to the chores next time to keep us entertained.
- **Collecting doggie-doo.** Buy clear plastic gloves at the dollar store, in packs of 100, and

kids will get a kick out of wearing them for picking up doggie-doo. *Make a game*: whoever collects the most poop in their trash bag wins "relax time" and gets out of the next chore...setting the dinner table.

Lifestyle Tips

- **Rewards for efforts.** Every day I hear myself tell my kids 'If you finish your homework by 4pm and do all your chores, you'll earn a reward.' Now I apply the same theory to myself! The main reward for me is feeling proud, which is timeless, and my kids seem proud to have a strong mom who can set up and take down our campsite single-handedly. But sometimes that just might not be enough, so having a back-up reward like a brownie sundae truly does the trick!

- **Get up and stand up.** I get up from my chair each hour, as I work. I'll go to the farthest bathroom, deliver a message by hand instead of emailing or run outgoing mail to an official blue mail box instead of using the red flag on my mailbox. If you need motivation to do this: a bowl of M&Ms in another room helps me get up from my office more often, with an allotted five M&M's per visit.

- **Practice good posture.** I envision having a malt ball or pile of cotton candy on top of my head that I must keep from falling! Other times I stand up tall and pretend there is a balloon on a string tied to my rib cage up through my neck and out the top of my head.

- **Keep house temperature cooler**. It saves money, conserves energy, and keeps me moving to stay warm. My thermostat is set to 62° F.

- **Shop for exercise gear.** Exercising provides mental happiness, and shopping for gear makes me excited to be up on the latest trends. Good gear makes me want to wear it to get out!

- **Get a dog.** Even on blustery days, my two dogs need to get out. In terrible weather, without dogs, I would never go out. But getting out in strange weather is beautiful. You get to see things like ethereal mist, beautiful wind, and crisp cold. A beautiful way to take a quick, healthy break!

- **Subscribe to a fitness magazine**. I leave them by every toilet and flip through them when sitting in the bathroom. I'm always reminded to try a new exercise or a new recipe. It's also easier to take in one bite of information at a time, as opposed to reading and trying to internalize an entire magazine all in one go.

- **Bookmark websites and blogs that educate and inspire you**. Here are a few of mine:

  www.goalsfortheweek.com
  A stay-at-home mom sets weekly goals for her different life roles and takes on triathlons.

  www.Hungry-Girl.com
  A blog that showcases and reviews the newest, tasty low-cal foods.

  www.Eatbetteramerica.com
  A great collection of easy recipes.

- **Perform actions of strength**. For example, I'll go camping for only one night which requires a lot of physical strength to set up and take down the tent and gear quickly! In another example, on a smaller scale, I pull my stomach in really tight as I refill ice cube trays with my purified water dispenser and as I carry them to the freezer. Doing things like that all day, engage my muscles and help me use what I consume! I want that cookie after dinner!

- **Race to and from places**. My kids love to play this with me. The airport is a great place for this. We race to the moving platforms, one of us hops on, and then the others see if we can beat the one on the platform to the end. This way we're active before sitting for a long period. We also run from the trampoline to the sink to wash hands before dinner.

- **Start small and follow through.** When I find myself annoyed at a chore, I come up with a game to push me through it or a reward for trying, and attack one chore at a time. When choosing the sock drawer to on focus, if I do extra sorting like underwear and bras, I'll get a bonus pat on the back. When I set expectations low in some situations, I'll get to meet and exceed them!

Diet Tips

- **Energy bars on-hand in two places: the car and my purse**. I always have a backup so I don't start opening boxes of cookies at the grocery store. Although, I still might be guilty of that!
- **Eat protein at every meal.** Protein keeps me fuller for longer. So when it comes time for sweets, I don't gorge!
- **Leave a full glass of water out** on the counter or desk, so it's ready to drink.
- **Split dinner** with a friend and save room for dessert.

- **Hard boil 6 eggs once a week.** They're the easiest source of all essential amino acids in the egg white.
- **Suppress hunger or boredom with exercise and water.** Next time a hunger pain surfaces, drink a glass or water and do three minutes of movement like marching in place, moving arms in big circles, doing 120 sit-ups, or running up three flights of stairs. Then wait 15 minutes. If still hungry after that, then eat! If the feeling passed then maybe it was at an unnecessary habitual time that could be broken. Every month I seem to have to play this game to retrain my mind's response to my stomach's misfired cue, to match my caloric needs.
- **Chew gum.** Gas stations make me smile, because while the gas is pumping, I get to check out the latest gum flavors! I'll have great breath and clean my teeth in between sweets.
- **Fast.** Seasonally, for just one day, I drink water, tea, and vegetable juice. It makes me feel lighter and it jump starts my short-lived healthy streak.
- **Make exceptions every week.** For example, I adjust food intake. I'll only eat a small, high-protein breakfast, skip lunch, and forgo snacks, if I know I'm going out for wine, salad, a full dinner and dessert later that evening!

- **Don't deprive**. Usually, when I deny myself what I'm craving, I end up eating it anyways, so sometimes I just skip a meal and enjoy whatever it is I'm craving. If I only eat an amazing piece of homemade cake for dinner, I make sure to take vitamins and exercise.

- **Track calories**. I approximate that running for 10 minutes burns 100 calories, and that walking for 10 minutes burns 50 calories. I log my time spent walking and running. I also keep a mental log of the obvious sugar and alcoholic indulgences. I try to match the exercise that same day or first thing the next morning to use any stored sugar as fuel!

Fitness Tips

- **Leave running shoes (and swimsuit for me) in the car, and music player in purse.** Occasionally I'll pull over when driving and run 20 minutes out and back. This is always refreshing to see the different neighborhoods and landscapes. It's like eye candy!

- **Keep a gym class or pool lap time schedule** in car glove box. Whenever I'm out I'll try fit in a workout, especially since I already have shoes and suit in the car at all times. In case I have unexpected errands come up and need to run out, and forget to check the schedule before I leave home, I can make sure I don't miss an opportunity by being able to check the schedule while I'm already out.

- **Keep all workout clothes in one drawer.** Socks, bras, shorts, shirts, bands, hats, workout plans or books to reference. One spot makes it super easy to get ready without wasting a second of your day! In the morning, when making breakfast, I can run from the kitchen to the bedroom, get dressed, remind myself of the workout I want to do, and return to open the waffle maker.
- **Lay out gym clothes the night before**. If it's in plain view, I'll use it right away.
- **Change up the exercise.** Instead of just walking or running steady, I add skipping, side steps, or trotting backwards for 40 seconds, about six to eight different times into my run. I'll do my weight workout in reverse order or look up a new exercise for triceps and change the move in the workout. This keeps things fresh and interesting.
- **Write down exact time.** If I haven't made an exact start and end time, it doesn't motivate me to do it. I can find a million things to do *that need to be done*, so I need a start time. On Sunday nights, I write down the times of a daily

workout schedule directly onto my calendar for each day.

- **Sign up for one exercise event each year.** Events make me more excited to exercise. Just one event a year keeps me thinking of the reason to maintain my strength. I enter a running race every year. So, sign up for a 5k race. Go ahead and try it. Search 5k races online, right now. Put the book down and challenge your fears! You can walk fast instead of run. Or you can run a quarter mile then walk another quarter mile, and continue in shifts through the whole race! Each race is always a fundraiser for something. By paying the entry fee you can feel good about donating! A race will also give you a good reason to go buy some cool new shorts! The power you get when training for something is unbelievable—it's great motivation!

- **Watch active people** on TV when working out. Program your DVR, TIVO, or MOXIE BOX to record shows that are fun, active and inspiring! My favorites are Wipeout, Minute to Win It, Survivor, Amazing Race, So You Think You Can Dance, America's Best Dance Contest or sports! ESPN has great for mainstream sports coverage and Fuel TV has amazing coverage of extreme sports like skateboarding, motor cross, surfing, biking, snowboarding, and X-games.

- **Create lists of friends for different activities.** I keep a list of friends with phone numbers next to my desk under different categories like walkers, tennis players, runners, hikers, yoga-lovers. That way when a spur-of-the-moment window of opportunity opens, I just call up a friend without having to think!

- **Switch iPods with a friend.** I highly recommend asking friends to switch! It makes me laugh (listening to some of the songs my friends chose) and gives me inspiration (some great songs that I've never heard before.) I've even cried on runs, when a friend's tune evoked a personal memory. Listening to their playlists is invigorating because it's unpredictable and makes for an interesting workout!

- **Do a burst of exercise** like a quick run up several flights of stairs, or a set of push-ups, as many times a day as needed for stress relief and distraction into present moment awareness. This helps me banish thoughts that dwell on future stress, and gets me back on track taking one task at a time.

- **Get dropped off to run home.** On drives home from errand running or vacations, my boyfriend will pull over 6 miles from our town to let me out. My kids wave at me running along the road. It's fun to reach home an hour later and see everyone there.

- **Bike around town for short errands.** Make it a family affair. Hop on a bike and go to the store, post office, pharmacy. You get the added bonus of reducing emissions and being eco-friendly! It's fun to think about what life would be like without cars!

- **Read Men's Fitness Magazines**. Try adding bits of their harder workouts into yours. I incorporate aspects of strength training from men's plans when mine feel easy or I just want to try something new.

15-minute Night Circuit

Once my kids are in bed, I have a positive routine that keeps me active. I do a 15-minute circuit as I start watching TV. It's restorative and engaging. It increases mobility, flexibility and metabolism. Do each of the 15 activities for 40 seconds and then rest for 20 seconds. (See 'Night Circuit Poses' on page 56 in Appendix.)

1. March with high knees. Hands behind head, knee touches elbows.
2. Cat and dog yoga moves. On hands and knees, swing torso down, looking up, and then round your back up, looking down. Repeat.
3. Downward dog. Palms on floor, arms straight, head looking down, buttocks up towards ceiling, legs straight, feet shoulder width apart, heels stay down. It's like an upside-down 'V.'
4. Wide-straddle squat and hold.
5. Downward dog, again.
6. Wall sit-ups. Place buttocks against wall, legs up on wall, lay on back.
7. Runner's lunges. Lunge forward with left leg, keep left knee beyond ankle, keep right leg straight back, and have both arms pointed straight up to the ceiling.
8. Wall sit-ups, again.
9. Runner's lunges, again, this time with the right leg.
10. Wall sit-ups, again.
11. Arm circles, forward.
12. Wall sit. Place back flat against wall, sit with knees at 90 degree angle, keep feet flat on floor, and hold.
13. Arm circles, backwards.

14. Laying torso twist. Lying down, hold top leg over the bottom leg at waist level. Hold 20 seconds each side.
15. Flat-back foldover. Both arms out straight. Bend at waist with flat back and straight legs, and place hands on the edge of a counter, table or couch arm. Hold for one to two minutes. This is my favorite in the circuit—it really releases weight on my hips. It's so great that I do this one every day, actually, before bedtime.

Commercial-time Exercises

When watching TV at any time of the day, I do some moves during the commercials. Here are my 3 favorite moves.

1. Turn your head all the way to the right and left slowly 10 times.
2. Look at the ceiling for a minute. All day we look down at our computers so your neck muscles are thankful for the change!
3. Hold both arms straight-up to the ceiling for a minute. All day they hang down!

Stay Lighthearted

When I'm in a light-hearted mood, I'm much more able to have a productive life, as well as be less annoyed with anybody or situation.

Here are some tricks I do to get in a good mood:

- **Go to the bathroom**. My dogs run to me whenever I sit on the porcelain thrown and I pet them. They know it's the most opportune time for me to focus my attention on them. (Obviously we're not a close-the-door-to-pee family!) Petting them is cathartic. They are so simple. I imagine going into their heads and feeling their peace.
- **Pretend any chaotic, uncontrollable, annoying situation is part of a film set**. Any difficult situation I face, I simply imagine we're being filmed. I'm an actress, and these pesky people are in the film. They are not really trying to annoy me, in a personal way. They're just there because of the film.
- **Breathe in deeply through my nose** with eyes closed and out through my mouth with eyes open.
- **Fake problem**. This is the quickest and easiest to incorporate into my days. It's a phrase I use

to stop we-have-a-problem thoughts. Since those negative thoughts trigger uncomfortable emotions (and no one likes to feel miserable) I banish those feelings immediately by saying these two words—fake problem. I acknowledge that it's just temporary and can then focus on my health, my lovely family, my great circle of friends, and my good life. If all that's so great, who needs fake problems? They're not real anyway!

- **Perform one stretch**. Stop stressful thoughts with a favorite stretch. Mine is is waterfall yoga pose. Let your head hang down loosey-goosey and try to let go of all neck tension. The head rush from blood changing direction flushes away unwanted thoughts. Okay, maybe that last bit is imaginary, but visualizing it makes the stretch even more impactful.

Enjoy the Week!

I like giving days nicknames, it makes any negative connotations associated with the days much less powerful. Mondays are *Manic Mondays*. Then I have *Tread-water Tuesdays, Wonderful Wednesdays* (since it's the one day both my kids have no sports practices or music lessons), *Thankful Thursdays*, and (you guessed it!) *Fantastic Fridays*, which can also be *Fart-astic Fridays* if we ate mom's chili on Thursday. The last two are definitely my favorite weekday names. Then we have *Super-duper Saturdays* and *Sleep-in Sundays*. Ahh! Great, fun names make the week flow by in a wave of positivity and optimism.

Chapter Three:

Diet Tips and Tricks

I love sweets, especially after a good healthy meal. However I know I can't perform solely on sugar. I need protein, calcium, vitamins, minerals, fiber, and healthy carbohydrates along with any sugar! Overall I believe in health. I also believe that calories from any food are usable fuel. So my philosophy is to enjoy my food and balance out my next choices to feel good.

"What is patriotism but the love of the food one ate as a child?"

-Lin Yutang

Health Biography

I was raised with two extremes. My mom was very health conscious, though occasionally she would splurge on sweets. She played tennis weekly. Today, she's still a strong woman. When I was young, she subscribed to wellness newsletters from Stanford and UC Berkeley which documented new trends in medicine and health. I was fed liver and spinach when they were popular sources of iron. Then there came the years of carob when that was suspected to be better than chocolate. Along came the spoonfuls of oat bran when it was announced as something that would add years to our lives.

Candy was restricted at home. I attended the movies with plastic bags of raisins and nuts. But my best friend's house always had cookies and sweets, so I ate much more than my parents knew. (Looks like you can never stop a sugar lover!)

Every chance I got to make homemade cookies, I would. My mom also enjoyed baking, cooking and making dinners. One of her labors of love was making *polechinthas*, traditional Hungarian crepes, with the thinnest batter I'd ever seen. The patience it took to make 40 individual crepes, one by one was admirable. It was in retrospect, later as an adult, that I gained this admiration of her commitment and patience. I recall her standing at the kitchen counter for hours, dipping the crepe maker into the bowl of batter, swirling it around evenly, and waiting for the first signs of bubbles to remove it from the heat. As the stack of crepes grew I could hardly wait to fill them with sweetened cream cheese, top them with her homemade berry compote, and the finishing touch—powdered sugar. After my mom poured some sugar into a small metal strainer, I'd delicately tap and sift the fine fairydust-like sugar through it. It was as pretty as the first snowfall on a mountain.

My dad, on the other hand, enjoyed lots of comfort food like potato chips and sweets. But my mom made sure he ate healthy too. With my Dad, I experienced the delight of cafeteria buffets. He taught me how to use the soup bowl for my ice cream sundae which was much bigger than the little cups by the machine! He was also an avid runner. I remember his lean legs poking out as he headed off for a run. He'd do it all: easy, long, tempo, interval or hill runs.

Another of our beautiful baking traditions occurred on Christmas morning. My dad's mom, Grandma Baker, baked sticky buns every year and we'd wake up to a house full of presents and the aroma of cinnamon sugar. It's really no surprise that my maiden name is Baker!

So with influences from healthy eating to comfort indulgences, I saw how each one made each of my parents happy, and I emerged in between. Needless to say, that both of my parents, with their unique take on food, are alive and kicking!

In junior high and high school, my stay-at-home mom made sure I started the day with a nutritious breakfast. Then at school, I spent my $2 lunch allowance on ding-dongs, mini powdered doughnuts, greasy cheesy rolls, and tater tots. After school I played sports: tennis in the fall, soccer in the winter, swimming in the spring. I'd stay at school until 5 pm practicing sports. Thank goodness I'd always end the day with a well balanced dinner!

Many parents stress out over their kids nutrition. I say if you have healthy choices available at home, take a daily multi-vitamin, stay active and give some sugar-lovin', it's all going to be okay. I eat a healthy diet about 80% of the time, and I feel great! I allow myself sugar because that feels good too. I think if it were restricted from my life it would become a bigger obsession!

All in all, I try to have fun as I'm being responsible. I see myself as the main character in my life's play, amusing myself (and hopefully others) with my activities and sugar-filled moments! I try to lighten up, accept my choices, and then balance out my choices so I feel good. Sometimes balancing out my sugar induced choices involves a healthy streak, so read on...

Eating Styles

I cycle through different eating styles which relate to my eating companion (girlfriends, partner, and kids), my menstrual cycle, and other hormone issues.

I believe balance is the key to everything in life, diet included. People don't generally talk about balancing extremes, just trying to eat balanced meals every day. This, of course, is a good goal. But Native Americans and early settlers, for example, didn't eat perfectly balanced meals day in and day out. They'd eat only meat for months on end without the availability of fruits and vegetables in the winter months.

I applied this logic last 4th of July, when I accepted a request to be in our town's pie eating contest. I like firsts--trying new things is my cup of tea. And when you combine that with sweets, I'm in, no questions asked! Locally-made, world-renowned Olalaberry Pie? Sure, bring it!

I'm competitive, but I really didn't care how I fared. (Well, maybe I did want to beat a few people!) My eating strategy was to eat only the filling, which weighed the most, and it paid off. I ended up scoring 5th place when the pie pans were weighed, out of about 20 eaters! To balance everything, for dinner later that evening, I ate raw broccoli and snap peas with hummus and some plain meat. This way, I got all the categories of the food pyramid.

So, basically, pie contest or not, I tend to cut myself lots of slack. In the spirit of the early settlers, I don't stress out if my daily or weekly intake isn't perfectly in-line with the food pyramid or my physical activity. I never turn down a delicious homemade margarita or dessert at a friend's house. They put their time and energy into making it and part of eating good food is feeling the love that went into making it! Balancing out my choices so that I'm able to enjoy sweets is what keeps my mind engaged.

If I don't eat a balanced meal one day, I'll balance my choices, somehow, in the following days and weeks. Because I have lots of positive habits in place, this helps me meet my goals!

Here are some styles of eating that I find entertaining:

- **Mini good streaks**: My rewarding game is to eat healthy for three days and the fourth day I get to eat whatever I want.
- **Moderation**: Days include checks and balances of the food pyramid in my head. If I eat an apple fritter for breakfast, that's one fruit, one fat and one carb. So, I try to fill in the rest of the pyramid for lunch and dinner (read 'Food Pyramid Guidelines' on page 7).
- **Portion-size**: Focus is on the size of portions at meals. I'll likely eat one "fist-size" portion for breakfast, two portions for lunch and three for dinner.
- **High sugar consumption**: There are days when I eat more carbs and sweets than is needed for basic survival. So, swinging 180 degrees towards a really healthy diet makes up for it. When my mind settles, I go back to eating in moderation.
- **Healthy streak**: Eat the healthiest thing available wherever I am, no sweets. When at my hormonal best this is possible for 14 days. If I'm on a healthy streak, I try to beat my last streak and make it to 15 days. Hasn't happened yet, here's to working towards it!

- **Big dinner style**: Cut breakfast and lunch in half, no snacks, drink water to hold me over and eat a fulfilling dinner and dessert.
- **Eat like a child**: Eat when I'm hungry and eat slowly. Gosh, my kids eat slowly! They talk and talk and talk and if I didn't say, 'Hey, put something on your fork please and let's finish dinner,' they may just hang out at the table for an hour. The upside is: they're my best role models. When I act like them, I feel happy. How simple is that! Take more time at dinner. Eat slower, eat what you crave. I try to put 3 colors of food on their plate each meal. Many nights they'll eat them all, some nights they won't. I'm more consistent with my offerings to them for breakfast and lunch, than I am with myself. So why don't I just copy them all the time? When I do, I feel pretty darn good! This is when I start laughing at myself, at the irony of recognizing a perfect habit, yet not doing it. I chalk it up to my brain needs problems to solve—it's a fake problem!

I remember when my kids were in high chairs. When they were done, they just started smearing, poking and throwing their food. I can laugh now at how irritated I felt at their messiness and how annoyed I felt in having to clean it up. But all in all, I've forgotten the headache because it all turned out fine. Because, they did, after all, grow out of ending their meals in that way!

I think that's how all of life is: messy at times, but turning out fine.

Food Balance

Let's face it, everyone has to watch what they eat. Not many of us can eat whatever we want. It's a known fact that as we age we need less food because our metabolism decreases, which is a major bummer, since I'm constantly learning to cook and bake better!

Overall, I know what I've eaten in a day. I make educated choices to indulge in desserts, skip snacks or lunches some days, cut meal portions in half other days. I guess because I tend to enjoy a lot of variety, I have to keep better track. If you've mastered your diet and rarely get lured off track, this book probably sounds silly. But for those who need the flexibility and variety, having several guideline eating styles, like those listed above, will allow for changing things up while still staying balanced. Anyway, it makes it more fun for me!

Healthy foods boost immune systems, develop bones, increase blood oxygen, and flush out toxins. This is why I love healthy foods. I also love sweet foods because I enjoy the process of creating them—baking, tasting and comparing sweets. Just as a wine enthusiast appreciates varieties of wines and the art of winemaking, I love sweets and baking.

And as it turns out, certain sweets have healthy benefits too. Chocolate, for example, contains polyphenols, which act as antioxidants to help combat oxidative free radicals in our bodies! Chocolate has been shown to have 2x the antioxidant levels of prunes, which have among the highest levels of fruits. And a report from Harvard University found that people who eat sweets, including chocolate, appear to live almost a year longer, on average, than those who do not. Pharmacologists at the Neurosciences Institute in San Diego have also shown that eating chocolate unleashes cannabinoids in the brain, which make us feel happy. Learning these facts helped me feel a lot better about including bits of it in just about anything. Researchers at UC Davis found that 1.5 oz of milk chocolate had similar antioxidant properties as a 5-ounce glass of red wine.

Personally, I feel like it's better to eat sugary sweet things and counterbalance that with health, versus eat a lot of sugar and doing nothing to help your body, or deprive oneself of all sugar and binge eat with guilty conscience. I really do advocate health and also advocate acceptance of sugar in my diet.

Occasionally blending health into my desserts or baking recipes fulfills both of my requirements. Engaging my left brain to modify ingredients and include different portions makes me feel smart like some sort of kitchen scientist! What will happen if I add a package of chopped spinach, use milk instead of water, and add a scoop of protein powder with an extra egg yolk to the box brownie mix? (It actually tastes pretty similar, surprisingly.) How will this pumpkin muffin batter turn out if I smash in half a cup of tofu, add some flax seed and an extra egg? (It turns moist and tasty too!)

Food has a history. When I bake and eat I delve into some subliminal connection to this food history. My foods and my eating habits don't spring out of nowhere, but rather they've developed over time, throughout my life. The memories, the love and the good old fashioned effort of my family and friends emanate through their baking and sharing. It seems unrealistic to strip myself of these beautiful experiences and cut out sugar completely.

There are times where I've reached my caloric necessity or I'm driving 5 hours to see my family, and need something to fiddle with. Sugar-free gum or Ice Breaker Sours help satisfy my sweet tooth. I also get the added bonus of not having to worry about brushing my teeth afterwards!

Get Your Fluids

Did you know your brain is 75% water? So, slight dehydration can cause headaches and worse. Water, water, water is all I can say. Two cups before each meal, one in between each meal and one at bedtime. That's my goal.

I read once that people mistake hunger for thirst. So I tried to be conscious of this; when I thought I was hungry, I drank water, and indeed it actually was true! My displaced feeling of thirst, or what I was interpreting as hunger, would go away with a glass of water. Every time I'm hungry I drink a glass of water or tea and it helps curb my appetite.

I drink V8 regularly for 2 servings of veggies and only 70 calories!

Hot cocoa is the perfect night time drink. It's warm and chocolaty—which is just plain delicious. And it's also kind of healthy! I usually make mine with two tablespoons of cocoa, two tablespoons of sugar, and one cup of skim milk. The total calories equal 150 per cup.

I love tea! Add a little Coffee-mate to any tea and it tastes like a cookie! Also, if you're a tea-lover, try cookie-flavored black tea by Lupicia—it's my new favorite.

I rarely drink juice or soda because I get more enjoyment from consuming baked goods and desserts. Calorie for calorie, I'd just rather sink into a slice of chocolate cake than drink a glass of soda.

And, boy, do I love smoothies! When overripe bananas get to the point when they won't be eaten, I peel and freeze them to use later. Mix one frozen banana, half a cup skim milk, four ice cubes, half a cup of water, one scoop of vanilla whey protein powder and two tablespoons of peanut butter for a delicious drink. This clocks in at about 400 calories. Substitute a cup of blueberries for the peanut butter, and this will bring you in at 300 calories.

Vitamins & Supplements

Here is what I take with my breakfast:

- Multi-vitamin for women
- Calcium, magnesium, zinc, and vitamin D (all in one pill)
- Omega 3 and 6 oils (in two different pills, from flax and fish oils)

As soon as I feel a little sick, I take an Airborne tablet or a powdery vitamin packet with water for a vitamin boost.

For sore muscles, adrenaline pumped days or if I start to feel a little sick, an Epsom salt bath works wonders. Toss two cups of Epsom salt into a warm tub, and soak for 20 minutes while listening to some mellow tunes. Try it out—it's the perfect ending to a hectic day. If curious, search "health benefits of Epsom salt" on-line and read about it's many benefits to the body. Epsom salt is made up of both magnesium and sulfate, which as it turns out, are easier to absorb through our skin vs. a supplement. So, take an Epsom salt bath, and reap the benefits ranging from relieving pain or muscle cramps, to flushing toxins, to improving nerve function and circulatory health, to relieving stress and migraines.

~

For more information on how to integrate a
healthy diet into a busy life, check out
Got Sugar? Recipe Companion.
It's filled with time-saving tips, kitchen guides,
and delicious, quick recipes for
meals, and of course, sweets!

~

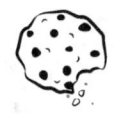

Chapter Four:

Thoughts on Exercise

Exercise burns. Every day, when starting out for the first five to ten minutes, my muscles hurt. It'll be like that until I'm warmed up. I might struggle at first but I keep going. Soon the exercise itself is rewarding enough that there's no need to search for external motivation. And man, does that last set of strength training hurt! But that's not a bad thing because it keeps me in reach of my goals. I know from experience —like after losing all strength and endurance from time off with injuries or pregnancies—that it's always easier to keep up than catch up.

I've trained for years to stay strong and maintain or increase endurance, and completed two marathons in 2009-1010, qualifying for Boston Marathon in 2011. I play co-ed baseball Monday nights two Seasons per year and women's soccer on Sundays. I also competed in the ABC obstacle-course game show "Wipeout" in June of 2010 and won my episode (#303 Anderson Can't Dance.) Bottom line, once I designed and committed to a plan that worked for me, I have felt so motivated to continue since I'm enjoying the benefits of being strong. (I outline the four plans I rotate between in my Workout Companion Book.)

Oddly enough, by stressing my body with exercise, I feel relief! It helps me get away from life when it overwhelms. Exercise calms my mind and I focus better afterwards with less stress. Exercise releases endorphins, which are known to alleviate mild depression. And the physical exertion itself helps me sleep more soundly at night! These reasons are good enough to make me love exercise, but there's more: when I work out, guilt for eating sweets is minimized.

When it gets tough, I still press on. In these cases, even if I don't run or lift weights as hard as I have in the weeks prior, I'll go through the motions at an easier lever and complete the work out in the allotted time. It's my main positive habit that keeps me grounded—so I never stray. I'll never say that I'm too tired for a workout, or that I'll try to make up with extra time tomorrow. On tough days, I'll still exercise, but I'll do it at a lower intensity. I feel good knowing that I didn't bail out. So although I didn't go all out, my confidence is still boosted. Amazing how that works! Just the pride in having exercising boosts my mood and makes me feel good about being strong!

Now that I've built some stamina over time, my legs, feet, tendons and joints have adapted. So I'm able to sustain my workouts more easily before tiring!

"The pessimist sees difficulty in every opportunity. The optimist sees the opportunity in every difficulty."
-Winston Churchill

Exercise Goals

I strive to maintain mobility, flexibility, and strength in my physical health. Since those three things matter to me, I feel happy working out.

A primary goal is to stay challenged and entertained with my workouts, since I get bored easily. Any diet or exercise regime gets boring. So, I change my schedule four times a year to hold my interest in the game (see 'Seasonal Workout Guide' in *Got Sugar? Workout*

Companion). I also tell myself really important things to keep motivated (see 'Play Games' in *Got Sugar? Workout Companion*).

Though there's definitely something to be said for routine, too much routine makes for a rigid and mundane program. If you aren't flexible, your workouts could get boring and you run the risk of losing interest and motivation. If you're program is too easy, you'll never stay in shape. So it's great to have a foundational structure in which you can easily flex and adapt.

Another goal of mine is to complete an efficient workout: get a good exercise session in the least time. I achieve this by alternating between muscle areas. Previously, I was doing three repetitions of triceps, resting, and then moving on to doing three repetitions of abs and resting again. I was resting for longer in between each set of repetitions, because the muscles hurt from using them three times in a row, and I wasn't able to do as many reps because they were exhausted. By doing what I call a rep-rotation, in which I exercise four different areas in immediate succession, I increase my momentum because I alternate muscle work and can work each area harder with less rest between those reps. (read 'Strength Training Workout Guide' in *Got Sugar? Workout Companion* for more.) I designed this program for myself when the many other methods didn't hold my interest.

> *"I haven't failed, I've just found 10,000*
> *ways that won't work."*
> -Thomas Edison

Visualize!

Each morning I visualize my strength and it makes me smile! If I exercise, I fulfill my goals, and fulfilling goals makes me happy! Visualize yourself doing the work, visualize yourself enjoying the work, and visualize yourself achieving your goals. It creates a positive, can-do mindset, as well as simply motivating you to get started on whatever stands before you.

Say Yes

I try to say yes to everything my kids ask me to play, with a hidden goal to raise my heart rate by playing with them for 10 minutes. If we're on the floor playing kitty, I'll hold a lower pose to work my arms as I make a bridge they can crawl under. If we're on our trampoline we'll see who can do 10 jackknife jumps in a row without falling over. We all try. Falling over and over as we play is all part of the fun, it's hilarious to cheer each other on! Then, when I get back to chores, like fixing dinner or paying bills, that great mood will have carried over. Bursts of action at random times, like playing with my kids, boost my level of playfulness, which keep me young at heart and makes me happy.

"Don't be afraid to go out on a limb. That's where all the fruit is."
-H. Jackson Brown

Why Not!

Another game I play is the 'why not' game. It's invigorating. Just saying 'Sure, why not!' is kind of like saying yes, but it's much more fun. When friends ask me to do things I've never done before like sailing, playing hand ball, helping set up for the school play, mountain biking in an unfamiliar area, I'll give it a try!

Applying this theory socially can really help you challenge your fears. Like doing karaoke—does that activity scare you? Why not just give it a try and see how it goes! The activity and the company are always rewarding (if nothing else, entertaining for your friends and you conquered a fear!)

When a friend asked me to join her on a night run, with a new head light strapped to my forehead, I said, 'Why not!' The experience was great—we saw a few deer, a raccoon and many birds!

When an instructor corrects my position, I don't take it personally, I'm receptive. People might give me advice when they know something I don't. Since it might work, I just say, 'Why not?!' and I'll try it out.

Exercise Tips

Here is a collection of random thoughts pertaining to exercise:

Try running random distances, called *fartlets* in running circles. I do this each week. I'll sprint to the end of my street, for example, or I'll sprint to a car, or I'll race to the mail box across the street and back.

Do twists and turns and lunges to different drawers as I unload the dishwasher. Or try timing yourself to see how fast you can unload it, and then try to beat it next time.

Do a short fast workout if you're short on time. Sprint for 20 seconds and walk 40 seconds, ten times to get your heart beating fast during a workout. Or, run for 15 minutes hard. That's better than walking for 15 minutes, especially if you like to eat sugar like me!

Get a gadget or app. *Fitdeck* Mobile on Blackberries or Fitness Builder on iPhones both offer exercises organized by targeted body areas. It's easy to keep finding new exercises so you don't get bored.

Get a head light so you can run earlier or later, to fit more into your busy day. They usually run about $20, and it's awesome entertainment! I turn my head left, right, slightly up, slightly down to see what I can light up in my path. Pretending there might be a cool animal just around the corner keeps me on my toes, staying ready to sprint away from it if necessary.

Enlist the '40-second on, 20-second off' rule everywhere! As I do laundry, I lift the liquid detergent in my right hand for 40 seconds while loading with my left hand. When volunteering at the grammar school, I park down the street and mini-skip backwards for 40 seconds to the entrance. I pull in my stomach for 40 seconds many times a day, even as I sit in my chair typing this!

Take the stairs. When I'm with my kids, we push the elevator floor button inside and then jump out to run up the stairs. We find it hilarious to see if we can beat the elevator to our floor. If we're stuck waiting for an appointment, we'll go up and down the stairs three more times together and time ourselves. We have fun betting on how much faster we can do it the third time.

When I'm being environmentally aware, I teach my kids that omitting the elevator timing game makes it an eco-friendly choice.

When flying solo, I like to see how well my strength training is working and I trot up the stairs. If I'm really in pain, I'll know that I probably need to work on my quads and do some extra bursting moves!

Exercise in random places. When I walk my dogs to the park, I'll do some yoga moves while they sniff and explore. I'll stretch, move from downward dog to cobra five times, and finish off with some warrior lunges. Initially I was uncomfortable outside at a public park. But after doing it a few times, and having people smile at me, it's made me happy that I challenged my fears and with my physical effort too!

Play with or near kids. Sometimes I grab my kid's skateboard or scooter and just go back and forth in the driveway, or I'll jump rope for 5 minutes while they are outside playing next to me. I wrestle with my son. I get goofy and dance around to some good tunes with them!

Own a big trampoline! I jump four to five times a week with my kids. I try to jump hard for a full minute without stopping, five different times. By jumping in the late afternoon I get an extra mini-burst of feeling strong!

Do micro-exercises while sitting in the car, watching sporting events, or waiting at the doctor's office. Performing these mini-moves twice a week challenges my mind to remember how many sets I did before getting interrupted. It not only gets you moving, but it also makes the time fly by!

Micro-exercises

I aim to do each move for 40 seconds, 3 times. I pulse them to the beat of the music!

- **Butt cheek clenches**: I make up variations like double-time for 8 beats, on the beat for 8, double-time for 8, on beat for 8, double-time for 8, and that's 40 seconds up!
- **Leg clenches:** Tighten tops of upper leg to the beat of the song.
- **Hand clenches:** With hands on the wheel at 2 and 10 o'clock, tighten fists into a clench.

- **Elbow squeeze**: With hands on the wheel at 2 and 10 o'clock, squeeze elbows in towards each other. Pulse or hold in as long as you can.
- **Toe scrunches:** These help build arch strength. You can do them while in cruise control in the car, or while sitting in a chair waiting.
- **Toe tapping**: This builds shin strength. You can also do these while in cruise control in the car, or while sitting in a chair waiting.
- **Heel raises:** These work your calves. Do these while in cruise control in the car, or while sitting in a chair waiting.
- **Tighten inner thighs**: Put a book, bottle of water or whatever item in between legs and hold.
- **Kegel muscle tightening:** Do this to the beat of the music!
- **Neck resisting**: Push on each side of head above ear, and resist. Push back against headrest, push on forehead with one hand. These are four different positions that are great to alternate and hold.
- **Waist wiggle**: Tighten stomach and move waist side-to-side to the beat.
- **Pull stomach in:** Flatten your back against the seat and pull your stomach muscles in.

- **One arm punch**: This is great to do to a rock song. Do it hard, so you feel it! It'll make another driver smile at you!

Structure is good, but occasionally toss out the workout plan! Do something new or different, faster or slower. It's great for mental health as well. For example, during the summer when I swim more, I'll drop the arm portion of the weight sets in the same week. Think of ways to change the exercise, while keeping in mind what muscles you want to work to keep a balance of arms, legs and core.

I try to keep doing more active things every day, not less. This way my body has a reason to use the sugary things I consume!

Injury Prevention Ritual

One of the most important things about getting healthy, is staying healthy. To do this, you need to stay injury-free. Injuries hurt, they zap time, and with an injury I can't move around as much. This means, I have less opportunity to use up the energy I've consumed.

So, each morning, to gear up for a day of movement, I perform a mini warm up. It's like a little injury prevention ritual that I do before I get out of bed. Do each of the following for 20 seconds:

1. Roll ankles.
2. Bicycle legs.
3. Straighten legs, flex and hold them up to the ceiling.
4. Slowly open and close legs for easy inner thigh and hip movement.
5. Hip stretch, crossing left leg over the right, grab left knee with right hand and hold. Then switch.
6. Sit up on bed side and roll neck. Look up, down, left, right.

Then when I stand up I've got some juices lubricating my joints and I'm ready for more movement.

Also good posture means better alignment and less chance of injury from favoring a side. So when you sit in a chair at work, try not to lean one way or the other. Sit straight and engage your back and stomach muscles to hold your torso erect.

And finally, to prevent injury, I <u>don't do the same thing two days in a row</u>. Different exercises stimulate different muscles, and there'll be less chance of overusing them and causing injury!

I do what works for me, modifying moves or positions to keep going. Variety is great! If my hip hurts, I'll skip parts of the workout that use my hip and focus on things that don't use it: I'll do more core and arm work until it's healed. I keep exercising but I modify the movements. Sometimes to prevent injury, I need to go at a slower speed.

And don't forget, drink water! Water lubricates connective tissue, which helps prevent injury!

Always remember to focus on where you're going, instead of where you've been!

~

For more information on workout tips
that inspire, check out

Got Sugar?

Workout Companion next!

It's complete with body areas,
exercise guides, strength training
suggestions, and annual
workout plans.

~

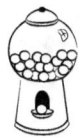

APPENDIX

Night Circuit Poses

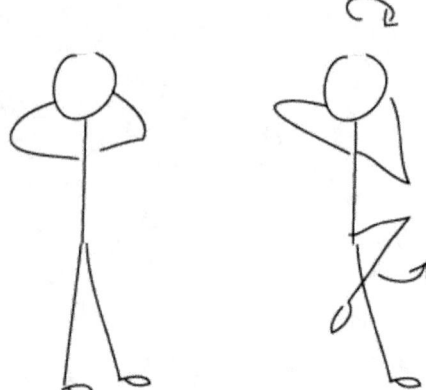

1. March with High Knees

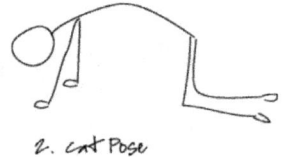

2. Cat Pose

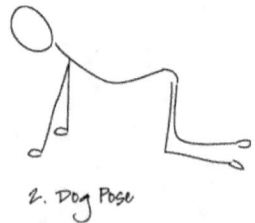

2. Dog Pose

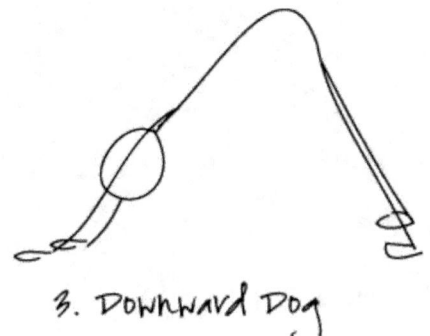

3. Downward Dog

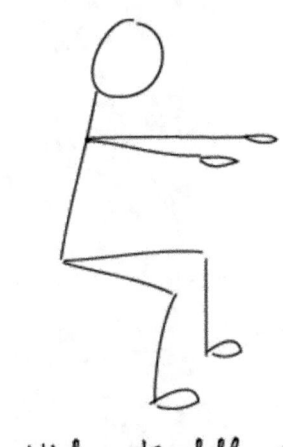

4. Wide-straddle Squat

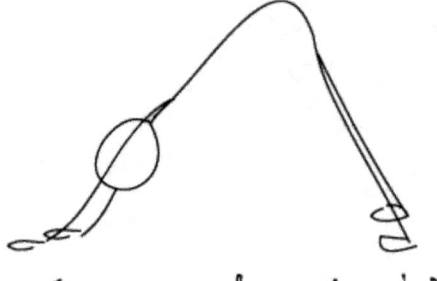

5. Downward Dog (again)

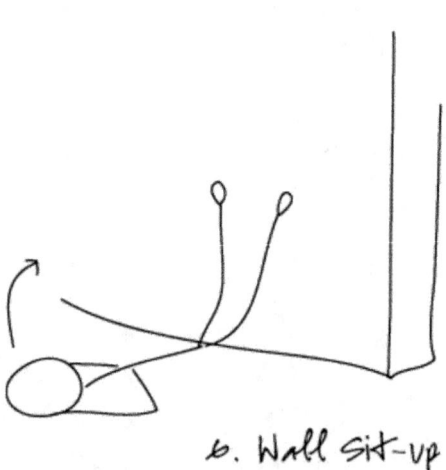

6. Wall Sit-up

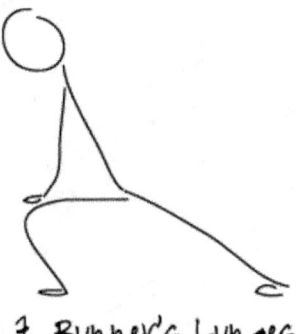

7. Runner's Lunges

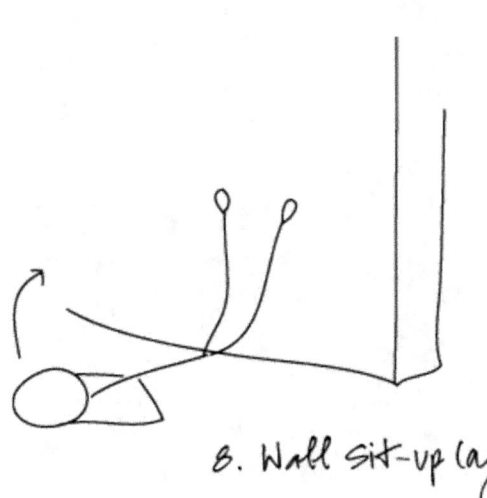

8. Wall Sit-up (again)

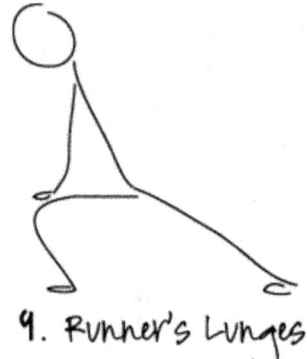

9. Runner's Lunges

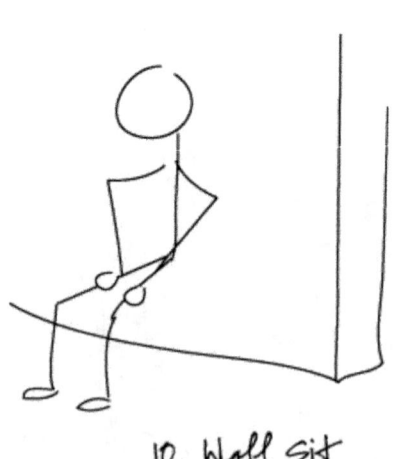

10. Wall Sit

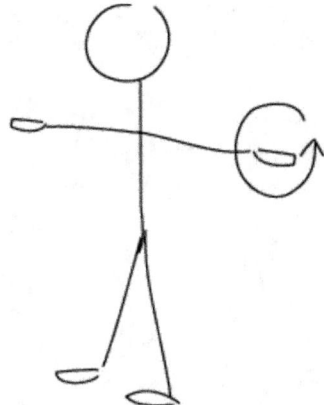

11. Arm circles (forward)

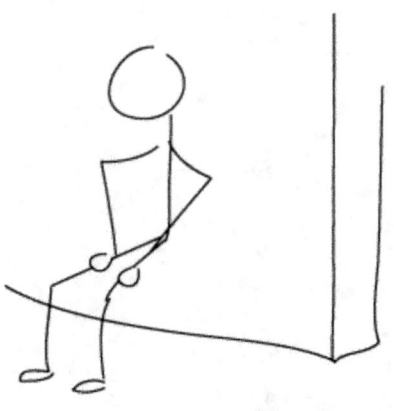

12. Wall Sit (again)

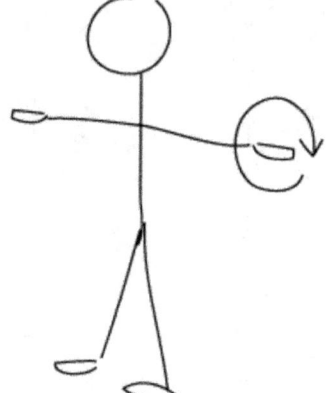

13. Arm circles (backward)

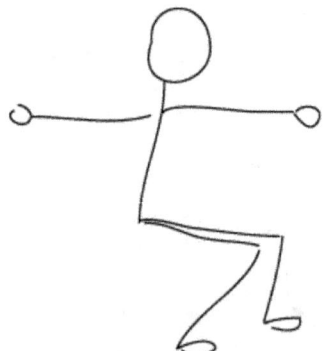

14. Lying Torso Twist
(aerial view)

15. Flat-back Foldover

Book #2

Got Sugar?

Workout Companion

*The Sweet Guide
to Fitness and Well-Being*

Debbie Markham

Note

The information in this book is believed to be accurate and true at the time of printing. The author can not accept any legal responsibility of liability for any errors or omissions that may be made nor for any inaccuracies nor for any harm or injury that comes about from following ideas in this book.

Comments welcomed:

debbie@functionablyhappy.com

Table of Contents

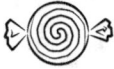

INTRODUCTION

This book for is for those who love to live life sweet. Now if you read my first book *Got Sugar?*, you know what I'm talking about. I'm just an average girl who loves staying balanced, healthy and fit, and I also love my sugar. Try to take my cake and you're in for a world of trouble.

Living life sweet isn't just about the sugary goods that I love to bake and eat. It's about making the most out of life. As a busy entrepreneur and single mom, I wanted to do it all without compromising in any arena. Over the years, I've mastered my own way of doing it all and enjoying it too. I love making the most of time with my kids, I love managing my own business, I love staying active and trying new sports, and I love ducking into the kitchen to round up a batch of sweets for family and friends. Through all of this, I've gathered up some of my life's philosophies—ranging from balancing and time management to staying healthy in spite of my own sweet tooth. These philosophies and a focused mind-set have helped me squeeze all the best out of life. And that's why I say my life is sweet, through and through. As I always say, there's always a way to have your cake and eat it too.

While I'm running my business or spending quality time with my family, I'm always thinking of healthy ways to satisfy my active, competitive spirit. I've created a great foundational exercise plans as well as some crazy, fun ways to staying healthy while managing a busy schedule. Beyond the workout tips, I also offer some foundational knowledge on staying healthy, perfecting form, and preventing injury.

When compiling the original *Got Sugar?*, I realized I didn't want to have a recipe-cum-workout book in my workout bag. I just wanted workout tips when I needed them, where I needed them, with no extras. I've now made *Got Sugar? Workout Companion,* so that you can have a little workout guide by your weights or in your drawer of workout clothes.

Learn about how to integrate a workout plan that works with your busy life. Because after all every girl deserves to do it all and enjoy the sweet life!

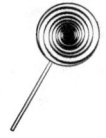

Chapter One

Foundations of a Great Workout Session

Breathe Right

When I'm exercising, whatever the workout might be, I create a calm within my storm. The storm is my physical stress, I'm working hard to move my muscles and pump up my heart rate. But through all this energy, I keep my mind clear as I focus on breathing.

In order to increase endurance, it's helpful to focus on something else and tie your breathing to it. When I run I have a 3-2 breathing rhythm. It matches my foot steps hitting the ground: I begin to inhale on my right foot, continue to inhale on my left foot, finish the inhale on my right foot. I then begin to exhale on my left foot, and finish the exhale on my right foot. When I'm sprinting a 2-1 breathing rhythm works better. Two breaths in, one breath out. Inhale on my right foot, continue to inhale on my left foot, and then exhale on my right foot powerfully! For swimming I breathe every three strokes. In yoga, breath is timed with the moves. While kayaking, I breathe in and out with each paddle. I learned each of these breathing rhythms by simply trying them out as I began a new activity. Try out these breathing patterns for these activities and make up your own breathing rhythms for any activity not listed here.

The Shoe Trick

I alternate between two pairs of workout shoes to prevent injury. When you use your workout shoes that inner foam compresses. And if you don't give the foam time to relax and decompress it can wear out quickly. Worn-out cushioning leads to an uncushioned impact as foot hits a surface as you run, jump or bike. This uncushioned impact can result in muscle damage or tendon wear. To avoid this, give you shoes time to regenerate their inner cushioning.

Warming Up is Key

This warm-up circuit can last for 2-5 minutes. In order to get my muscles warmed up and my joints moving, I complete 20 seconds each of the following activities, rotating them until my warm-up is complete:

- March in place
- Step side to side and touch one foot to the other
- Roll wrists and ankles
- Easy jumping jacks
- Stretch and hold various arm areas that feel like a good stretch
- Stretch and hold runners lunge for each leg
- Lean over touch shins or floor
- Trot in place

After you've completed your warm up, all the joints are lubricated and are less prone to injury!

Play Mind Games

Mind games amuse, distract, encourage and propel continuation of movement!

I'm a runner primarily, so I play tons of games throughout each run. When I run on the sidewalk, alongside a main road I have different games than a trail. For 15 seconds, I'll leap big strides as I run, trying to land each foot in 1 square of sidewalk, not touching the cracks. I play that game a few times until I've exhausted the benefit from the challenge.

Then for 20 seconds, I'll run with my heels touching my buttocks. After that I might *zigzag fast around* man holes, gas or water cutouts. I might do tiny leaps over cracks, gum marks on the ground, basically anything that I can jump over. I pretend there are secret drivers on the road scouting out great running form, looking for a runner to appear on the next cover of *Runner's World Magazine*. After a series of games like theses, 20 minutes will have passed and I'm feeling pumped! I play games with myself for other workouts as well. Other games I've integrated into my running sessions include:

• I aim to reach the halfway mark of my workout session. Then when I reach it, I tell myself everything is easier because I'm closer to the finish!

• When bursting, I imagine that I'm going for the finish line or the world record. This encourages me to go as hard as I can for 20 seconds.

• I pretend every runner or biker that I pass is my long-lost relative or friend. This fuels excitement when I see them, and then the adrenaline rush propels me to continue.

Positive Talk

Whenever I work out I try to give myself a pep talk that a supportive coach or workout trainer might give. These constant words of positivity not only help me continue during a difficult section of training, but they also build an optimistic mind-set that is key for exercise. Anytime you approach a workout, a can-do spirit is essential. Even if you're not feeling up for a challenge, try out some positive talk. I find that if I start thinking motivating things to myself, I'll soon internalize it, and simply start focusing on the exercise benefit ahead of me.

Here are some example pieces of positive talk that I integrate throughout my workout sessions:

• When I'm running a hill, I'll tell myself, 'I'm earning the downhill.'
• I always say to myself, 'I can do any exercise, any movement, anything for another 20 seconds.' This helps me finish a session without giving up, I end up pushing harder with more energy and spirit.
• 'I am a good role model for my kids.'
• 'I am strong, I can do it!'
• I never say, 'I wish I hadn't worked out today.'

Keep up the positive talk and your thoughts will be positive to.

Stretching

Stretching is important for a cool down.

At the end of my workout I stretch for 10% of the time I worked out. For example: I'll stretch for 2 minutes after a 24 minute workout. I tend not to stretch during my workout session because it relaxes me too much!

I once read that 20 seconds is the perfect length of time for stretching, and that stretching for any longer wasn't found to be that much more beneficial. So, I stretch 20 seconds per muscle. At the end a 40-minute session of swimming for example, I'll do 4 different upper body stretches, 2 different core stretches, and 6 different leg stretches. That's a total of 12 stretches, and at 20 seconds each, I end up stretching for 4 minutes, 10% of my original workout time. It might be difficult to integrate at first, but after trying it out a few times, you'll get into a pattern of stretching.

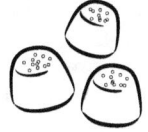

Chapter Two

Breaking Down the Basics

All About Aerobics

Aerobic workout improves endurance.

Each week, for 2-3 of my workout days I choose one of the activities: swimming, cycling, running, inline skating, kick-boxing, doing the elliptical trainer, rowing indoors on a machine, stepping on the stair-master, or following a home exercise video.

All these are aerobic workouts, geared towards strengthening your heart and improving the oxygen system of your body. When your heart is stronger, it can pump a higher level of blood and deliver more oxygen rich blood throughout your body!

To grab some ideas for aerobic workouts search online. For example, to find some swimming workouts, type 'swimming workouts'" into the search bar. Your internet browser brings up many sites to reference from easy to moderate. A great DVD I watched to pump up my swimming sessions was *Total Immersion Swimming*. It was the best investment I made to improve my swimming form. I grew up swimming on a swim team and this DVD still helped!

Researching and improving "correct form" for any exercise maximizes your health benefits and minimizes your risk of injury. Since it's always great to actually see the form, as opposed to reading about it, search for some photos or videos.

After practicing your form, if needed, for whatever aerobic workout, start making up games! Games for aerobic workouts will help push you forward and motivate you to keep moving. Here are swimming games to play: swim 500 yards made up of 10 fast 50s (swimmer's talk for 10, 2-length segments) on the 1 minute 40 seconds. Then swim 5-100s (5 x 4 lengths of the pool: 1 length Right arm only, 1 length Left arm only, 1 length kick, then the last length Pull with both arms - no kicking.) Set time limits for doing things like: swimming 5-100m IMs (or individual medleys made up of butterfly, backstroke, breaststroke and freestyle) within 10 minutes (try to do each 100 in less than 2 minutes.). When I'm out of ideas, I swim a pyramid: 1 lap fast, 1 lap slow, 2 laps fast, 2 laps slow, all the way up to 5, then back down to 1 lap fast, 1 lap slow.

The same types of games, which play with varying speed and setting goals, are adaptable to any type of aerobic workout. If you're excited to tackle biking, start out with basic workouts by searching online 'bicycle workout' or 'biking workouts.' Later on don't forget to add your own games to these workouts for fun! Insert sprinting 8-10 different times, to different points (like the first piece of trash you see on the road, or to the next telephone pole up the road, or to the first manhole you come across) throughout your workouts for a challenge with entertainment.

When following my workout plans, on the aerobic days, feel free to integrate the type of aerobic activity that gets you going! All the guidelines for running (like pushing hard for 18 minutes, going easy for 12 minutes, or sprinting for 40 seconds, or types of mental games mentioned above) can be applied to any aerobic activity.

Relax with Yoga

Yoga relaxes, strengthens and focuses your mind, body and spirit.

The more often I practice yoga, the more I hear and embody the words of the yoga instructors. Instead of just doing the poses for strength and maintenance of joint mobility, I also do yoga for mental meditation to help relieve stress and promote acceptance. Caring, nurturing words are spoken by the instructor while I focus on my yogic position. Yoga challenges my mind and body to hold unique poses that distract me from all other thoughts. It is a beautiful workout that I integrate weekly.

Many times I invite friends to a yoga class and their responses are 'No, because... 'I haven't done it in so long' or 'I don't really know the moves' or 'I can't balance well and will be self-conscious.'

In response, I just want to say that no one in any yoga class cares if someone loses balance, falls down, or sits down and don't participate for moments. No one cares if someone wears old running shirts and shorts. Everyone in yoga class is focused on their own state, their own body, their own meditation—not anyone else's.

That's the beauty about yoga. It's truly an independent and non-competitive activity. Instructors are there to help us feel good about ourselves. Bottom line, it's too much effort to feel anything else BUT my own stuff: thoughts bubble up and I try to let them go, while I feel unusual muscles being used and I attempt to focus on the desirable slow breathing technique using my nostrils. Everyone's focused on themselves so no one attending a yoga class for the first time, or after a long time needs to feel self-conscious.

One day a week, usually on a Sunday, I practice yoga or follow a Pilates DVD. Since they take too long for my busy weekdays, I usually save them for the weekends.

When first starting out with yoga, I felt guilty and selfish for leaving my one-year-old daughter for classes. Needless to say, it was traumatic for us both. She'd scream and cry, and though it hurt, I stuck to my positive habit and would leave for class. Each time I completed my yoga class, I felt so refreshed. I was rejuvenated and excited to return home. Then when I'd see my daughter smiling, doing well without me, I felt happy about sticking to my workout goal.

On the other hand, when I'd stay at home to exercise with a DVD, at first, I was continually approached by my kids. But I stuck with my exercise goal, as I explained my efforts to my kids. By kindly stating that I needed to take some time to focus on exercising, my kids eventually learned the routine. I'd say, 'Mommy's exercising. Come and join me or I'll help you when I'm finished.'

By letting them know that while I'm busy they're welcome to join I reinforced bonding as well as promoting positive, healthy habits. And by letting them know that I'll be available afterwards, I let them know that I'm still here for them. Though they were reluctant at first, they soon accepted that I focused on working out during workout hour and they learned not to interrupt me anymore. Occasionally, they love to join in and tout that they 'do yoga' or 'do Pilates.'

For busy women who balance family life and professional life, finding time to do time-consuming meditative exercises like yoga and Pilates might seem impossible. Understand that your kids can do great without you for an hour or two, and that you'll feel happier and rejuvenated after your workout so that you'll be able to tackle your busy days with a smile.

Vital Strength Training

Strength training builds and maintains your muscles.

Two to three days a week I do strength training, which is a weight and resistance workout. It not only strengthens muscle (which burns more calories than fat), but it also increases bone density, strengthens the heart and increases metabolism for the rest of the day!

My strength training days involve rep-rotations of exercises for 4 different groups: arms, legs, core, and bursts. Each set of reps last for 40 seconds with 20 seconds rest in between.

If this sounds completely confusing and you want to put down the book right now, don't! Just breathe—it all gets spelled out in an easy-to-follow way. The next section will break down the possible exercises within the various strength training groups (see **Part III: Strength Training Groups**), while the section after next will present simple rep-rotations as a sample strength training workout sessions (see **Sample Strength Training Session** in **Part IV: Strength Training Workout Guide**).

My personal philosophy is to maintain my muscle mass, since I've achieved a desirable strength, not build it. So I lift a manageable weight. The weights I go between are a pair of 5 lb. dumbbells and pair of 8 lb. dumbbells. If you're looking to tone up or maintain your shape, lift a similar light weight. When you start lifting heavier weights, this will build muscle.

In order to gear up mentally, I prepare myself for some muscle burn. When my muscles start to burn at 20 seconds, I push myself through the burn. Tell yourself that you can do it for 20 more seconds, because you'll get to rest for 20 seconds. This way, you'll be motivating yourself to keep up the 40 seconds work for all your strength training exercises!

The Basics of Bursts

Bursts increase agility and stability.

Bursts are segments of increased effort or speed in any workout. I include one rotation, a full 40 seconds of bursts, in my strength training sessions. These inserted bursts produce powerful action and develop muscle power. Some examples of my bursts are jumping jacks, two foot hops, and toe taps. Find some more great idea for bursts in the next section (see **Group 4: Bursts**, in **Part III: Strength Training Groups**). Bursts are included in my strength training rep-rotation, which is completed two to three times a week.

You can also integrate bursts into aerobic workouts. Some sample aerobic bursts include 20-second sprints or super-fast skipping. Bursts integrated into your aerobic workout will help increase strength, speed, and stamina. For example, after warming up for a mile, I burst for 20 seconds out of a normal pace, then recover at a normal pace for 40 seconds. I complete this pattern of bursts 8 more times. It always surprises me that I actually do have reserve energy and I can sprint after an easy run. After all, different muscles are used for sprinting than running at a steady, normal pace.

Bursting can help prevent injuries by building muscles for power that long, slow work cannot.

Chapter Three

Strength Training Groups

This strength training guide is divided into four groups, the first three are body areas and the last group is bursts which incorporates various body areas. In each body area, there's a list of various exercises that you could integrate into your strength training days. Because these don't require large spaces or specialist equipment, you can easily do them at home or work in between tasks.

Group 1: Arms (four areas)

1. Biceps (front muscles of upper arms)

Dumbbell Curls

With weights in each hand, elbows bent at waist and palms up, lift the dumbbells toward your chest. Be controlled when lowering to start position. Keep upper body still, let biceps work.

Narrow Push-Ups

Hands are directly under shoulders and elbows touch waist when lowering.

2. Pectorals (chest muscles)

Laying Dumbbell Press

Lay on bench (or ottoman), weights in hands just above shoulders, palms face feet. Press weights straight up over your collar bone. Lower down, elbows end below level of bench.

Wide Arm Push-Ups

Arms out 1-2 feet out from the sides of torso, at shoulder height. I generally complete these using my knees, or try 8 full body push-ups first, then drop to my knees for the last 10.

3. Triceps (back muscles of upper arms)

Chair Dip

Get a chair (or bathtub edge) and face away from it, arms behind, knees bent, lower body down then back up.

Kickback

Split leg stance, lean forward with a flat back. With weights in both hands, keep arms pressed against torso. Start position is with bent elbows, holding weights chest height with palms in. Move by unbending and bending at elbows. Keeping elbows at waist, focus on dropping forearm and pressing all the way back, until arms are straight, as high above your back as possible. Bring back in and repeat. Alternate arms or try both at same time.

(Triceps continued)

Lying Triceps

Lay on the floor, legs straight up to ceiling. Weights in hands straight up to the sky over chest. Bend at elbow bringing weights next to ears.

Side Push-up

Lay on your side, legs together. Using the one arm closest to the ceiling, push down into floor to raise shoulder up off the ground, lower back down.

4. Deltoids (shoulder muscles)

Sitting Dumbbell Press

While seated, hold a weight in each hand at shoulder height, feet on floor. Press up and in above your head, slowly lower.

Shoulder Flies

With weights in hand, arms at a 90 degree angle bent at waist, palms facing in, lift forearms up from waist and out to the side up to shoulder height, then slowly lower back to your sides.

Side Raises

Standing up, feet shoulder-width apart, arms at sides, hold weights with palms facing inward. *Keep arms straight* and lift out to side, up to shoulder level. Lower slowly back to your sides.

Upright Row

Hold weights in hands, starting with straight arms at sides, with palms facing back. Raise elbows so that weight are up in front, under your chin. At the finish position, elbows are at eye level. Lower and repeat.

Group 2: Legs (four areas)

1. Calves (muscles from back of knee to heel)

Toe Raises

Stand on the edge of a step with balls of your feet. Lower heels slightly below step level, rise up onto tippy-toes.

Heel Walk

Lift toes off the ground and walk on your heels. This not only works calves, but also helps ankle strength too.

Angled Toe Raises

Stand with feet shoulder-width apart, toes pointing out towards the corners of the room. Holding weights in straight hanging arms, rise up on your tipsy-toes as high as possible, pause for 1 count and lower.

2. Gluts (buttock muscles, from pelvic bone to top of upper leg)

Fire Hydrant

Start on hands and knees, lift bent leg outward until thigh is at same height as body. Hold for a second, repeat other leg.

Kick the Sky

Start on hands and knees, lift bent leg up backwards and kick up towards the sky with your heel.

Glute Bridge

Lie with your knees bent, with a book or object between them. Squeeze your glutes and raise your body by lifting your hips off the floor and upwards. Lower your hips 1 inch from the floor, but don't touch it.

3. Hamstrings (muscles on back of legs from buttocks down)

Heel Dig

Lay on back, legs bent at 90 degree angle with heels on a chair. Push down into your heels and raise hips off floor. Bonus: Try Heel Digs simultaneously with Laying Triceps for maximum efficiency!

Stability Ball Calf Curl

Lay on back, legs bent at 90 degree angle with calves on a ball. Arms lie on floor next to body. Push down into your palms and raise hips off floor as you bend your knees to bring the ball towards your glutes. (ending with soles of feet on top of the ball.) Extend legs and repeat. Bonus: Glutes.

4. Quads (front of thigh)

Goddess Hold

Straddle your legs for a wide squat and hold arms out to your sides at a 90 degree angle, palms facing your ears. Hold the squat and feel the goddess in you - strong and calm, breathing deeply through your nose, and radiant with positive energy!

Wall Chair

Sit with back against a wall. Hold the position for a period of time.

Squats

Feet shoulder width apart, squat down as far as you can go, stand up. Play squat games: like pulsing down for 3 mini squats, then standing, then pulsing again, or like lowering slowly for 2 counts and then up for 1 count. Bonus: these also work your glutes and hamstrings.

Multi-tasking Moves

(calves, hamstrings, glutes and quads)

These are very efficient ways to exercise all 4 muscles of the legs. Great for those who are short on time! If you only have time for one leg exercise, do one of these lunging moves for maximum muscle group strengthening.

Forward Dumbbell Lunge

Hold a weight in each hand hanging straight down, pull shoulders back, tighten your core. Keeping your chest up, take a giant step forward so that your knee touches the floor. Push back to standing position. Alternate legs. These work your glutes, abs, calves, quads, and hamstrings.

Lunge and Turn

Grab a 10-12 lb. weight and hold it in front of your chest with both hands. Step forward with 1 foot into a lunge, then turn your torso towards the lunging leg, to twist. Push back to standing position. Alternate legs. These work your glutes, abs, calves, and quads. Bonus: Core

Walking Lunge

Walk forward with lunges. Take large step with right foot, lowering into a lunge. As you come up onto your forward-placed right foot, immediately take another lunge with your left leg. Holding weights adds intensity. These work your glutes, hamstrings, calves, and quads.

Group 3: Core

The core includes <u>two main groups of muscles</u>: **back** and **abdominal**. A strong core will contribute to being better at any activity as well as generally improve your posture and overall well-being. Great posture will help keep your body aligned. Core muscles help support the spine, hips and mid-section. They also enable flexing, extending, and rotating.

Back Muscles (two areas)

1. Traps (muscles along upper spine, help shoulders)

Alternating Dumbbell Row
Bend forward at hips. Holding weight in each hand, let arms hang straight down with palms facing thighs. Pull back by bending elbow and raising upper arm toward middle of your back. Alternate arms.

2. **Lats** (muscles on either side of the back, stabilize torso)

Back Extension

Lie down with stomach on the floor, legs straightened and arms against your side, with palms facing in. Using your back muscles, not arms, raise your torso up off the ground. Pull your torso up as far as you can, remembering to tighten your buttocks and concentrate on working the lower back. Hold this position for about 3 seconds. Lower, then repeat. Alternatively, you can just hold it as long as you can.

Abdominal or Stomach Muscles (three areas)

Be sure to work on all 3 abdominal muscle groups each week: one rotation each of <u>upper abs</u>, <u>lower abs</u> and <u>obliques</u>. If you develop your abs unevenly (like only doing crunches) your sides and lower abs which support your spine become weak.

<u>Fast sit-ups</u> recruit more muscles than slow ones, reports the Journal of Strength and Conditioning Research. So remember to mix it up and do at least one set as fast as you can.

1. Upper Abs (muscles above the belly button)

Regular Crunches
Lie on your back with legs bent, curl shoulders off the floor.

Shoe Touch
Lie on your back with legs bent, feet on floor, and arms on floor straight. Crunch up and try to touch right hand to right shoe, lower down,

then left hand to left shoe, and down. Bonus: these also work your obliques.

Reach for Feet
Lie on your back with arms raised, and straight legs aimed towards the ceiling and split like the letter 'V'. Raise your torso with your abdominal muscles, reaching with both hands to the left foot, then lower, then to the right foot, then lower (or legs together and just reach straight to toes.)

Mountain Climber
In push-up position, quickly alternate raising 1 knee at a time towards chest. Bonus: these also work your arms and legs.

V-ups
Lie on your back, legs straight and arms stretched straight above head. Simultaneously lift legs and torso, as you reach arms towards your toes. Using all the core strength you can muster, keep legs and back straight, creating a strong 'V' position.

2. Lower Abs (muscles below the belly button)

Criss Cross

Lie on your back, with arms at your sides, hands under buttocks, and legs raised off ground by 1 foot. Cross right over left, left over right, repeating the movements over and over again. Bonus: these also work your inner thighs.

Laying Plank

Lie on your back, with arms at your sides. Lift feet and shoulders a few inches off the floor to be in a wide 'V' position. Hold this position.

Seated Crunch

Sit on the edge of bench or bed. Bring knees to chest then extend straight. Bonus: these also work your quads.

Bicycle 1

Lie on your back, with arms at your side. Lift legs straight out off floor and towards chest. Alternate legs. Bonus: these also work you quads.

Hip Hip Hooray!

Lie on your back, with legs straight up to the ceiling. Lift hips and lower body off the floor as high as possible, with heels still aiming towards the ceiling. Lower, then repeat. Keep legs straight and use lower abs to control this small movement.

Pull-up Crunches

Lie on your back, with legs lifted 1 inch off the floor. Pull both knees at the same time up towards chest. Extend legs back out, then repeat. Bonus: these also work your quads.

Plank

Lie on your stomach, place forearms on the floor. Lift up torso while supporting weight on forearms and toes. Keep legs extended and straight, and keep torso straight and still. Hold this position. Bonus: these also work your arms.

Step Downs

Lie on your back, with hands under your lower back. Lift both legs up to bend at a 90 degree angle. With a slow controlled movement, straighten and lower one leg so that heels almost tap the floor. Bring leg back up to 90 degree angle and then do the other leg. Continue to alternate legs. (or to mix it up, lower both legs together a few times.)

Exercises for <u>both upper and lower abs</u>

The Boat

Sit up with knees bent towards chest. Balancing on tail bone, lift legs so that your straight torso and legs create as close to a 'V' position as possible. Keep arms outstretched to either side of your knees. Hold this position. Bonus: these also work your quads.

Bicycle 2

Lie on your back with hands lightly placed behind ears. Lift chest up, then twist to touch right elbow to left leg, and twist to touch left elbow to right leg. Continue alternating this movement. Bonus: these also work your quads.

Roll-ups

From a standing position, drop to the floor by bending your knees and rolling backwards onto your back. Pull knees up towards chest into a curling position. Engage your stomach muscles to quickly roll up from standing position to curling position. From the curling position, lean forward to roll out of curling position to standing position.

3. Obliques (muscles on the sides of torso)

Rainbow Legs

Lie on your back with arms out to the sides and legs bent at a 90 degree angle. Dip legs together to the right, not touching floor. Then bring legs back to the starting position. Dip legs together to the left, not touching the floor. Then bring legs back to starting position. Repeat these moves recreating a rainbow-like arch using your legs. For a harder workout: do with straight legs pointed towards the ceiling, dipping right and then left.

Cross Knee Crunch

Lie on back with feet on the floor, and knees bent and spaced shoulder-width apart. Curl shoulders off floor twisting torso right, back down, then left, back down, and so on.

Wall Twist

Lie on your back with buttocks against a wall and feet straight up onto the wall. Curl torso up and twist right, back down, then up and twist left, back down.

Side Plank

Lay on right side and prop yourself up on your right elbow. Raise your hips off the floor with a straight torso. Hold 20 seconds, switch sides for the left oblique. Bonus: these also work your quads. Variation: **Side Crunch** Lie on your right side with legs outstretched and hands placed lightly behind ears. Lift straight legs and crunch left elbow to touch top leg. Repeat movement on your other side.

Reach for Heels

Lie on your back, with legs bent so that feet on the floor are a foot away from buttocks. Reach with right hand to the right heel, then lower, then left hand to the left heel, then lower.

Group 4: Bursts

These exercises rev up your heart rate, strengthen many muscles at once and increase agility. They engage core muscles, increase stability in ankles, knees, quads and calves.

Straight Jump-ups
Jump straight up, hands reach for the sky, land as softly as you can.

Side to Side, Front to Back
Jump with feet together, side to side up over an object on the floor 10 times, then jump front to back over the object 10 times. Repeat.

Jump Up Stairs
Jump with both legs up 1 or 2 stairs, walk down. Repeat as fast as you can.

Jump Back
Jump backwards up 1 step (or up a curb) with both feet simultaneously, then jump down with both feet landing at same time. Repeat.

Skip High

Skip in place, or skip around in any direction, with knees as high as you can.

Tire Toes

Zigzag forward on the balls of your feet, like you are stepping into the center of tires on the floor, then backwards.

Circle Run

Run around an object on the floor, 20 seconds clockwise, then reverse. Keep legs low in an almost squat-position - go sideways, backwards, forwards. Remember to stay low.

Sideways Lunges

Start standing feet together and take a big step to one side, and lunge (making sure your knees are directly above your feet in the final low lunge.) Keep chest still facing forward, and keep your knee over your foot as you lower. Push back to standing, and then do a sideways lunge to the other side.

Alternating Toe Taps

Place a soccer ball on the floor 1 foot in front of you. Place your right toe on top of the ball, then switch feet quickly and tap the top of the ball with the left foot. Repeat.

2 Feet Hops

Stand up and hop forward, moving around the house!

Toggle Taps

Raise left arm and right leg, then bounce to land on right leg, simultaneously raising right arm and left leg. Now start toggling between sides. When left foot is down, left arm is up, and switch. The faster, the better!

Standard Jumping Jacks

Stand with hands down at side and feet together. Simultaneously, jump so that feet are apart, beyond shoulder-width, and throw hands to meet above your head. Repeat motions back and forth. Throw in a clap over your head if you're feeling extra energetic!

Chapter Four

Strength Training Workout Guide

Create Strength Training Sessions

My strength training sessions are filled with repetitions (or reps) of a selected exercise from the extensive list in the previous section. I, then, rotate these reps in order to get a full workout for each area of my body: arms, legs, and core. To finish, I'll complete a series of repetitive bursts. I call these my 4-minute rep-rotations. I'll complete three 4-minute rep-rotations to complete one set. And I'll do two or three sets for each strength training session. In total, this equals a great, well-rounded 24 or 36-minute workout.

Here are directions to help you craft a strength training session:

Group 1: Arms
Choose an upper body muscle from biceps, triceps, deltoids, and pecs. Then pick a corresponding exercise like Curls, Chair Dips, Flies, or Wide Push-Ups. Do this exercise for 40

seconds, then rest for 20 seconds, equaling a total of 1 minute.

Group 2: Legs

Choose a lower body muscle from quads, hamstrings, calves, glutes. Then pick a corresponding exercise like Squats, Heel Dig, Toe Raises, Bridge, Lunge, or a Multi-Leg exercise. Do

this exercise for 40 seconds, then rest for 20 seconds, equaling a total of 1 minute.

Group 3: Core

Choose a core muscle from your back or abdomen. Then pick a corresponding exercise like Crunches or Back Extension. Do this exercise for 40 seconds, then rest for 20 seconds, equaling a total of 1 minute.

Group 4: Bursts

Choose a bursting move like Jumps, Hops, or Skips. Do this exercise for 40 seconds, then rest for 20 seconds, equaling a total of 1 minute.

Each new exercise starts when the second hand hits the zero second mark, and ends at the 40 second mark. You rest for 20 seconds, until the second hand hits zero again. Rotating between group gives each muscle time to recover before you work it again.

With this rotation, I find that I'm able to really focus and push hard on one exercise, knowing that I will get to rest that muscle for three minutes as I work the rest of my groups.

Feeling energized? Try working 45 seconds and resting for only 15 seconds. Short on time? Rest for 0-10 seconds between reps and shave 2-5 minutes off your total workout time. When I only have 20 minutes, I know I can do the 2 sets (normally 24 minutes total) in 20 minutes if I don't rest between 40 second intervals. I'l just roll one into the next without stopping, increasing the cardio component and fitting in a balanced workout very efficiently.

These moves can also be done on various gym machines. But the real beauty is all of these moves can be done at home or in the office with two hand held weights. And professional women with kids know this kind of flexibility is key for maintaining a healthy lifestyle while juggling a busy schedule.

I find that even when traveling, these are easy to do, so there's never any excuse to not be able to workout. In a hotel room, I can do lunges between queen beds as my kids sleep, or I can use the chair that no one sits in during downtime for my dips and heel digs. Basically you can do this routine anywhere!

When the last rep-rotation gets difficult, play games with yourself as described in Part I. Make your own goal to push through it. I like to chant, 'This rep is for my body, this one's for those brownies!' Then the next set I'll chant, 'This rep is for my body, this one's for that glass of wine!'

I sprinkle these strength training sessions 2-3 times a week in between my other activities, so that I get a balance of strength training workouts, muscle elongating aerobic workouts (like swimming or running), and muscle stretching and toning workouts (like yoga).

Sample Strength Training Session

On my strength training days I'll complete a session much like the sample on the following pages. I'll do two or three 12-minute Sets to complete a quick 24 or 36-minute workout.

Set 1

This sample 12-minute set focuses on deltoids, quads, upper and lower abs. This first set completes 3 reps of arms (deltoids), 3 reps of legs (quads), 3 reps of core (upper and lower abs), and 3 reps of bursts. Notice that the bursts aren't done right after legs. The core exercises are placed in between legs and bursts to allow your legs a full-minute of rest.

1st Rep-Rotation (4m)

1. **Arms, deltoids**: Shoulder Fly (40s)
   Rest (20s)
2. **Legs, quads**: Squats (40s)
   Rest (20s)
3. **Core, abs**: Elbow Plank (40s)
   Rest (20s)
4. **Bursts**: Jump Up Stairs (40s)
   Rest (20s)

2nd Rep-Rotation (repeat above, 4m)

1. **Arms, deltoids**: Shoulder Fly (40s)
   Rest (20s)
2. **Legs, quads**: Squats (40s)
   Rest (20s)
3. **Core, abs**: Elbow Plank (40s)
   Rest (20s)
4. **Bursts**: Jump Up Stairs (40s)
   Rest (20s)

3rd Rep-Rotation (repeat above, 4m)

1. **Arms, deltoids**: Shoulder Fly (40s)
   Rest (20s)
2. **Legs, quads**: Squats (40s)
   Rest (20s)
3. **Core, abs**: Elbow Plank (40s)
   Rest (20s)
4. **Bursts**: Jump Up Stairs (40s)
   Rest (20s)

Set 2

For the second 12-minute set choose different muscles. This sample set completes 3 reps of arms (triceps), 3 reps of legs (whole leg and glute), 3 reps of core (side abs), and 3 reps of bursts. After completing this set, you'll have worked out for 24 minutes.

1st Rep-Rotation (4m)

1. **Arms, triceps:** Chair Dip (40s)
   Rest (20s)
2. **Legs, whole leg and glute**: Walking Lunge (40s)
   Rest (20s)
3. **Core, side abs**: Cross Knee Crunch (40s)
   Rest (20s)
4. **Bursts**: Jumping Jacks (40s)
   Rest (20s)

2nd Rep-Rotation (repeat above, 4m)

1. **Arms, triceps:** Chair Dip (40s)
   Rest (20s)
2. **Legs, whole leg and glute**: Walking Lunge (40s)
   Rest (20s)
3. **Core, side abs**: Cross Knee Crunch (40s)
   Rest (20s)
4. **Bursts**: Jumping Jacks (40s)
   Rest (20s)

3rd Rep-Rotation (repeat above, 4m)

1. **Arms, triceps:** Chair Dip (40s)
   Rest (20s)
2. **Legs, whole leg and glute**: Walking Lunge (40s)
   Rest (20s)
3. **Core, side abs**: Cross Knee Crunch (40s)
   Rest (20s)
4. **Bursts**: Jumping Jacks (40s)
   Rest (20s)

Set 3

For a third and final 12-minute set, choose different muscles. This sample set completes 3 reps of arms (biceps), 3 reps of legs (calves), 3 reps of core (back, lats), and 3 reps of bursts. After completing this set, you'll have worked out for 36 minutes.

1st Rep-Rotation (4m)

1. **Arms, biceps:** Curls (40s)
   Rest (20s)
2. **Legs, calves**: Calf Raises (40s)
   Rest (20s)
3. **Core, lats**: Back Extensions (40s)
   Rest (20s)
4. **Bursts**: Tire Toes (40s)
   Rest (20s)

2nd Rep-Rotation (repeat above, 4m)

1. **Arms, biceps:** Curls (40s)
   Rest (20s)
2. **Legs, calves**: Calf Raises (40s)
   Rest (20s)
3. **Core, lats**: Back Extensions (40s)
   Rest (20s)
4. **Bursts**: Tire Toes (40s)
   Rest (20s)

3rd Rep-Rotation (repeat above, 4m)

1. **Arms, biceps:** Curls (40s)
   Rest (20s)
2. **Legs, calves**: Calf Raises (40s)
   Rest (20s)
3. **Core, lats**: Back Extensions (40s)
   Rest (20s)
4. **Bursts**: Tire Toes (40s)
   Rest (20s)

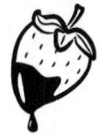

Chapter Five

Seasonal Workout Plans

Here are four seasonal plans to get you through an entire year. Busy women don't have much time to plan their workouts, no less an entire year's worth of comprehensive, holistic training. So these plans are great in that they offer some structure--a foundation or a starting base. You'll find that there's some variety thrown in to make sure you do all that your body needs in one week and through the seasons. Each season has a driving focus that will help push you through the workout weeks.

Despite the structure presented in these four workout plans, the rep-rotation exercises can easily be varied. If you're like me, you might get bored easily, and you'll be wanting to change the rep-rotations for each strength training day.

If you like to master a specific sequence, then you may enjoy working continually with the initial suggested rep-rotations. Either way definitely works! So find a groove that works best for you.

If you don't go to a gym, invest in two handheld weights for arm exercises. And if any of the following exercises or movements cause pain, simply don't continue.

To keep up my positive, healthy routine, I tend to workout six days a week. I start with a short warm-up and I cool down with some relaxing stretches. This is my positive habit, that I stick to, to reinforce a healthy mentality and a spirit of rejuvenation. In addition to these workouts, I walk my small dogs for 10 minutes each morning and evening. Two days a week, I do a 15-minute night circuit (see **Night Circuit** in *Got Sugar?*). I do micro-exercises two to three times a week in the car. And I regularly race around my house daily between rooms and chores (see **Exercise Tips** in *Got Sugar?*).

I usually choose Monday as my day off. Mondays are the most hectic, stressful days for me, with the start of the week, so it feels great to get a break and not exercise. I generally have more free time on Saturday and Sunday, so I always fit in a slower-paced workout on the weekends.

Taking 7 days *completely off* from working out, in between seasons, feels refreshing and is a fantastic reward for working 12 weeks in a row, 6 days a week! Give your body and mind the rejuvenating rest it needs to support you for the next 40-60 years. When I take time off, it feels weird at first, like I'm being lazy, then really great! I look forward to my seasonal breaks now. Knowing they are just around the corner keeps me committed to staying strong and less likely to skip days. After resting for a week, I'm itching to start a new seasonal workout plan.

Having the four different plans to look forward to, keeps me motivated and interested in working out. When I didn't have a yearly plan, I would randomly get burned out, not have an exact plan to reference, and lose momentum. Now, with 4 - 12 week plans, I know I can do 8 more weeks of any plan (since the first 4 weeks always go by fast.) Having goals of getting through each season with a new plan helps me stay focused, having a time frame of 12 weeks makes me try harder since I know the routine will end, and keeps my mind happy with the excitement of a week off and a change of schedule.

12 weeks of a seasonal plan with 1 week off, 4 times a year, equals 52 weeks in the year. Create your own program within this parameter to help yourself stay pumped up.

Spring Plan

The Six-minute Factor: Workout time goes up six minutes each day. Warm up 2-5 minutes (10% of workout time is my guideline.)

Monday
Day Off

Tuesday
Strength Training (24 minutes)
Do three 4-minute rep-rotations for the first 12-minute set. Then choosing different muscles, do another 12-minute set to complete the 24-minute workout. Cool down by stretching for 2 minutes. Do 6 different stretches, 20 seconds for each stretch.

Wednesday
Steady-pace Aerobic Workout (30 minutes)
Do a steady-pace aerobic workout and add 8 random lengths of sprinting. Make it fun! Sprint to the tree, to the curb, to a car, whatever. Do what makes you feel happy! Maybe you want to run 2 songs and walk 1. Or perhaps you want to throw in some skips every 2 minutes—believe me, it'll make the other runner smile. Cool down by stretching for 3 minutes. Do 9 different stretches, 20 seconds for each stretch.

Thursday

Strength Training (36 minutes)

Do three 4-minute rep-rotations for the first 12-minute set. Then choosing different muscles, do two more sets to complete the 36-minute workout. Cool down by stretching for 4 minutes. Do 12 different stretches, 20 seconds for each stretch.

Friday

Steady-pace Aerobic Workout (42 minutes)

Do a steady-pace aerobic workout, breathing a bit faster than Wednesday, but not out of breath. Cool down by stretching for 4 minutes. Do 12 different stretches, 20 seconds for each stretch.

Saturday

Easy Aerobic with Bursts (48 minutes)

Do a 20-minute aerobic workout at an easy pace. Then do eight 20-second bursts, trotting for 40 seconds after each. This is an 8-minute burst-and-trot sequence. Finish with a 20-minute steady-pace aerobic workout. Cool down by stretching for 5 minutes. Do 15 different stretches, 20 seconds for each stretch.

Sunday

Yoga (54 minutes)

Do a yoga class or follow a yoga DVD. Truly, I'm able to do any activity because of yoga—it keeps me flexible. If you really don't want to give yoga a try, then do a 40-minute aerobic activity with 14 minutes of stretching.

Summer Plan

The 24-42 Flip: Workout alternates every day between 24 minutes and 42 minutes. Every two weeks, flip the length of strength training days and aerobic days. This is a plan for four weeks. Do this plan three times and then you'll be set for the entire season.

Week 1 & Week 2

Monday
Day Off

Tuesday
Steady-pace Aerobic Workout (42 minutes)
Do an aerobic workout in which you're breathing a bit faster than normal, but not out of breath. You can always add random bursts of skipping, grapevine, or side shuffles to mix it up! Cool down by stretching for 4 minutes. Do 12 different stretches, 20 seconds for each stretch.

Wednesday
Strength Training (24 minutes)
Do three 4-minute rep-rotations for the first 12-minute set. Choosing different muscles, do another set to complete a 24-minute workout. Cool down by stretching for 2 minute. Do 6 different stretches, 20 seconds for each stretch.

Thursday

Steady-pace Aerobic Workout (42 minutes)

Again do another aerobic workout in which you're breathing a bit faster than normal, but not out of breath. Cool down by stretching for 4 minutes. Do 12 different stretches, 20 seconds for each stretch.

Friday

Strength Training (24 minutes)

Do three 4-minute rep-rotations for the first 12-minute set. Choosing different muscles, do another set to complete a 24-minute workout. Cool down by stretching for 2 minutes. Do 6 different stretches, 20 seconds for each stretch.

Saturday

Easy Aerobic with Bursts (42 minutes)

Do a 17-minute aerobic workout at an easy pace. Then do eight 20-second bursts, trotting for 40 seconds after each. This is an 8-minute burst-and-trot sequence. Finish with a 17-minute steady-pace aerobic workout. Cool down by stretching for 4 minutes. Do 12 different stretches, 20 seconds for each stretch.

Sunday

Yoga

No time limit on the yoga session because Monday is a full day of rest! If you don't like yoga, do a different kind of aerobic workout.

Week 3 & Week 4

Flip it! Now the 24-minute workouts are aerobic and the 42-minute workouts are for strength training.

Monday
Day Off

Tuesday
Strength Training (42 minutes)
Do three 4-minute rep-rotations for the first 12-minute set. Choosing different muscles, do two more sets to bring you to 36 minutes. Add 6 extra reps of your choice to complete a 42-minute workout. Cool down by stretching for 4 minute. Do 12 different stretches, 20 seconds for each stretch.

Wednesday
Steady-pace Aerobic Workout (24 minutes)
Since it's a short workout day, go easy for 4 minutes. Then do an 18-minute aerobic workout in which you're breathing harder than normal, but not out of breath. To complete do an easy 2-minute aerobic workout. Cool down by stretching for 2 minutes. Do 6 different stretches, 20 seconds for each stretch.

Thursday
Strength Training (42 minutes)
Do three 4-minute rep-rotations for the first 12-minute set. Choosing different muscles, do two more sets to bring you to 36 minutes. Add 6 extra reps of your choice to complete a 42-minute workout. Cool down by stretching for 4 minute. Do 12 different stretches, 20 seconds for each stretch.

Friday

Steady-pace Aerobic Workout (24 minutes)

Since it's a short workout day, go easy for 4 minutes. Then do an 18-minute aerobic workout in which you're breathing harder than normal, but not out of breath. To complete do an easy 2-minute aerobic workout. Cool down by stretching for 2 minutes. Do 6 different stretches, 20 seconds for each stretch.

Saturday

Easy Aerobic with Bursts (42 minutes)

Do a 17-minute aerobic workout at an easy pace. Then do eight 20-second bursts, trotting for 40 seconds after each. This is an 8-minute burst-and-trot sequence. Finish with a 17-minute steady-pace aerobic workout. Cool down by stretching for 4 minutes. Do 12 different stretches, 20 seconds for each stretch.

Sunday

Yoga

No time limit on the yoga session because Monday is a full day of rest! If you don't like yoga, do a different kind of aerobic workout.

Fall Plan

The AM-PM Split: Do 2 mini-workouts per day, one in the morning and one in the evening. Remember to warm up and cool down with each mini-workout.

Monday
Day Off

Tuesday
AM Aerobic Activity of Choice (20 minutes)
PM Strength Training (12 minutes)
Do three 4-minute rep-rotations for a single 12-minute set.

Wednesday
AM Aerobic Activity of Choice (15 minutes)
PM Strength Training (12 minutes)
Choosing different muscles from yesterday's strength training session, do three 4-minute rep-rotations for a single 12-minute set.

Thursday
AM Aerobic Activity of Choice (20 minutes)
PM Strength Training (12 minutes)
Choosing different muscles from yesterday's strength training session, do three 4-minute rep-rotations for a single 12-minute set.

Friday

AM Aerobic Activity of Choice (15 minutes)
PM Strength Training (12 minutes)

Choosing different muscles from yesterday's strength training session, do three 4-minute rep-rotations for a single 12-minute set.

Saturday

AM Aerobic Activity of Choice (30 minutes, or more since it's the weekend)
PM Strength Training (12 minutes)

Choosing different muscles from yesterday's strength training session, do three 4-minute rep-rotations for a single 12-minute set.

Sunday

Yoga

No time limit on the yoga session because Monday is a full day of rest! If you don't like yoga, do something active that elongates your muscles. Try to stretch longer.

Winter Plan

The Three-a-Week Focus: *Each strength training day focuses on a different group.* Since weather is less predictable for outdoor aerobic activity, I do this plan in the winter since it's indoors 3 days.

Monday
Day Off

Tuesday
Strength Training, <u>Focus: Arms</u> (24 minutes)
Do this 4-minute rep-rotation three times to complete a 12-minute set.

- **1. Arms,deltoids** (40 sec)
  Rest (20 sec)
- **2. Core, back** (40 sec)
  Rest (20 sec)
- **3. Arms, pecs** (40 sec)
  Rest (20 sec)
- **4. Bursts** (40 sec)
  Rest (20 sec)

Choosing different muscles, do another 4-minute rep-rotation three times to complete a 12-minute set.

- **1. Arms, triceps** (40 sec)
  Rest (20 sec)
- **2. Core, back** (40 sec)
  Rest (20 sec)
- **3. Arms, pecs** (40 sec)
  Rest (20 sec)
- **4. Bursts** (40 sec)
  Rest (20 sec)

Cool down by stretching for 2 minutes. Do 6 different stretches, 20 seconds for each stretch.

Wednesday

Steady-pace Aerobic Workout (42 minutes)

Do 42-minute aerobic workout in which you're breathing a bit faster than normal, but not out of breath. Cool down by stretching for 4 minutes. Do 12 different stretches, 20 seconds for each stretch.

Thursday

Strength Training, <u>Focus: Legs</u> (24 minutes)

Do this 4-minute rep-rotation three times to complete a 12-minute set.

1. **Legs, quads** (40 sec)
   Rest (20 sec)
2. **Core, abs** (40 sec)
   Rest (20 sec)
3. **Legs, hamstrings** (40 sec)
   Rest (20 sec)
4. **Bursts** (40 sec)
   Rest (20 sec)

Choosing different muscles, do another 4-minute rep-rotation three times to complete a 12-minute set. (see next page)

1. **Legs, calves** (40 sec)
   Rest (20 sec)
2. **Core, abs** (40 sec)
   Rest (20 sec)
3. **Legs, multi-muscle** (40 sec)
   Rest (20 sec)
4. **Bursts** (40 sec)
   Rest (20 sec)

Cool down by stretching for 2 minutes. Do 6 different stretches, 20 seconds for each stretch.

Friday

Steady-pace Aerobic Workout (42 minutes)
Do 42-minute aerobic workout in which you're breathing a bit faster than normal, but not out of breath. Cool down by stretching for 4 minutes. Do 12 different stretches, 20 seconds for each stretch.

Saturday

Strength Training, <u>Focus: Core</u> (24 minutes)
Do this 4-minute rep-rotation three times to complete a 12-minute set.

1. **Core, lower abs** (40 sec)
   Rest (20 sec)
2. **Bursts** (40 sec)
   Rest (20 sec)
3. **Core, multi-muscle** (40 sec)
   Rest (20 sec)
4. **Bursts** (40 sec)
   Rest (20 sec)

Choosing different muscles, do another 4-minute rep-rotation three times to complete a 12-minute set.

1. **Core, upper abs** (40 sec)
   Rest (20 sec)
2. **Bursts easier bursts like jumping jacks** (40 sec)
   Rest (20 sec)
3. **Core, obliques** (40 sec)
   Rest (20 sec)
4. **Bursts harder bursts like split jumps** (40 sec)
   Rest (20 sec)

Cool down by stretching for 2 minutes. Do 6 different stretches, 20 seconds for each stretch.

Sunday
Yoga (42 minutes)
No time limit on the yoga session because Monday is a full day of rest! If you don't like yoga, do something active that elongates your muscles. Try to stretch longer.

Book 3

Got Sugar?

Recipe Companion

Everything You Need to Satisfy a

Healthy Sweet Tooth

Debbie Markham

Comments welcomed:
Debbie@FunctionablyHappy.com

To Zoe and Nate, the best helpers to have around anytime, but especially when baking. And to the family and friends who have endured messes and flops, and countless new creations! Thanks for always helping me clean up.

Table of Contents

Chapter Seven:

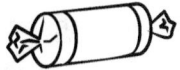

INTRODUCTION

As I admitted in my first book *Got Sugar?*, I'm a sugar fiend. I love to have my sweet treats. I love them so much, I'll make and eat them on a daily basis. But this doesn't mean that my health gets compromised and my time goes to waste as I indulge in these devilish treats.

I'm an average, modern girl who wants to make everything happen. I balance a full schedule of running my own business and taking care of my family as a single mom. Throughout my busy life, I want to make the most of time with my family as well as finding quality time for maintaining my health and cooking up some great memories in the kitchen.

Throughout these recipes you'll find loads of time-saving tips. We modern gals are rushed to no end. It's been great sharing tips with my own friends in order to learn and help each other make the most of our time. Now I'm really excited to share these time-saving strategies with you. From organizing your kitchen goods to cutting corners on recipes to make it work with your pantry, your time, and your taste—I've laid it all down here. With these time-saving tips, even the busiest woman will find a way to make a sweet treat for herself and her family at the end of a long day.

If you've caught my *Got Sugar? Workout Companion*, you'll know that I'm also very health-conscious. I care about staying strong and heart-healthy. This makes me feel rejuvenated, positive, and motivated throughout the day. My healthy ways, despite my love for sugar, do not stop at the kitchen door. I bring all my healthy ways down deep into the kitchen and into the mixing bowl.

You might be wondering how in the world has the love of sugar and the love of fitness wound up in one woman. Well, it's quite simple really. Many see them as totally opposite—which is why there are countless number of diet plans that don't allow women the pleasure of enjoying a treat after a meal. I don't see fitness and health as polar opposites to baking and eating desserts. With balance, healthy exercise habits, and a focus on getting all your nutrients and vitamins, you'll find that you can enjoy dessert and still be extremely healthy.

After all, food is an important part of our lives. Looking back on my childhood, I remember those stomach-warming meals that my mom used to cook up, or those treats that my best friends and I would enjoy in the summer sun. All the beautiful history of human life and culture are wrapped up in our recipes. From the smell of baking bread to the fun that my kids and I have when we're baking up a storm, food has a way of creating beautiful memories. I'm delighted to share this passion for food with my family and friends, as well as pass them on through this book.

Food is important for our bodies, our health, and our fitness. Those vital nutrients are key in building our muscles, keeping our brains bright and clear, and helping our young kids grow. There's a beautiful balance in this basic necessity and the creativity that goes into crafting a meal. The taste, texture, visual presentation—it's all a gorgeous part of prep time and meal time in my family.

As I look back on each of these recipes, I see how deeply woven they are into my memories, my relationships with friends and my good times with family. Recipe sharing is social—that's the beauty of it! Favorite time-saving meals, traditional family dishes, crazy dessert concoctions. All these great tips and secrets get passed around through friends and family, making each one of these dishes rich with love and sweetness.

As you take a look at these stories, tips, meals and desserts, I hope that you'll find some stories with which you can identify with and something new that can help you enhance your meals. And, be sure to find some time and some space in your heart to enjoy a sweet treat every once in awhile.

Part I: Kitchen Staples

These are staple items that I try to have on hand at all times. I keep the following list printed out and stored in my kitchen drawer. Each week, I just scan the list to remind myself of the staple items I want in my kitchen. Then with every shopping trip, I throw in some other essentials like seasonal fruit and veggies, bread, milk and cheeses.

Making your grocery list can be a positive experience, by turning it into a game. When it's time to start listing items, think...Do I need flour? What about tuna? If I guess correctly (before looking at the supply in my pantry or fridge) it's a bonus - I get happy! Creating a fun-spirited game in my mind around household tasks, like maintaining my kitchen stock, truly makes me a more optimistic, balanced woman. <u>Make your own list of essentials, photocopy it and keep it handy to make life easy on your brain each week!</u>

Refrigerator and Freezer Items

Eggs: These are rich in essential amino acids, vitamins A, B, D, trace minerals and antioxidants, and are one of the few foods considered a complete protein!

Ground Turkey: Lean meat allows more room for sweets.

Smoked salmon: Pre-packaged delicious smoked salmon can usually be usually found near the lunch meat or deli section.

Low-fat cream cheese and bagels: These go great with smoked salmon.

Low-fat Greek yogurt: This is so thick I really can't believe it's low fat! If you can find the Kigo brand Greek yogurt, you'll get a bonus side-car of honey that you can drizzle into the yogurt. So yummy, I promise!

Non-Fat cottage cheese: Great way to get protein - eat with fruit or atop a baked potato. Can blend it into a smooth consistency similar to sour cream or for a faux cheese cake!

Lemon and lime juice: Grab these in the plastic squirt bottles so you can save time squeezing. Good on on salmon, added to water, or included in Lemony Bars (page 37).

Hummus and pesto: Grab the tubs of freshly prepared hummus and pesto so you don't have to make it at home.

Garlic in a jar: Seriously the best time-saver ever. Love the taste it adds to your meals, hate the extra time it take to crush, mince, pulverize, as well as wash it from your hands.

Dijon mustard, soy sauce, and Italian dressing: These condiments are great to use for marinade and cooking sauce for fish and chicken.

Bacon pieces: Go for real bacon pieces, not those dehydrated, processed bacon bits. Add to eggs, baked potatoes, pasta, chicken casseroles, and salads. I usually find these in a big bag at Costco— the best deal! Or at grocery stores, you can find them near the salad dressing section.

Non fat milk and soy milk: Stay balanced by limiting your fat intake in your milk consumption. This gives you some room for desserts.

Fresh vegetables: Baby carrots, celery, cucumbers, broccoli and zucchini make super easy snacks (especially dipped in the next item!) and mixed greens for a salad. Beets are my new favorite side dish - rinse, cut tops off and wrap whole in foil and bake for 50 minutes at 300 degrees. Cut and serve as is, sweet tasting like corn with texture of a potato.

Frozen chicken breasts: Grab a giant value bag of chicken to get the most bang for your buck as well as saving time on eliminating trips to the grocery store. I get the Foster Farm packages of 12 breasts at Costco.

Frozen filets of fish: Again, try to grab a giant value bag of fillets. Many stores sell big bags of individually packaged filets.

Frozen blueberries: These are super-duper little nutrient-filled fruits. Grab them frozen and you'll get a better deal. They are just about the most versatile fruit - great for adding to pancakes, smoothies, muffins and yogurt.

Frozen vegetables: It's great to have vegetable back-ups when you might not have time to get the fresh stuff for evening meals. Spinach, edamame, green beans, mixed veggies, corn are some of my consistent favorites.

Frozen brown rice: Save tons of time by getting fully cooked bags of rice. You can find big bags of frozen rice at Costco or smaller sized bags at Trader Joe's.

Shelved Goods

McCormick recipe inspirations: These little cards give you a recipe and measured portions of spices that you can easily integrate into the recipe provided or into one of your own.

Seasoning Packets: Taco Seasoning, Mesquite Seasoning and Pesto Packets have enhanced the taste of my meals many nights.

Salsa, marinara sauce, diced canned tomatoes, tomato paste: All these tomato-based items are seriously essential. You'll always be able to create of improvise some dish.

Cans or jars of artichoke hearts: The raw stuff takes a bit of effort to steam and prepare. So grab the artichoke hearts that are already prepared – they're waiting to be let out of their container into your salads, sandwiches and meals.

Cans of different beans: White or pinto beans, kidney beans and black beans.

Soups: tomato, cream of mushroom, cream of chicken, broth: Any soup is comforting to eat as a light meal: soup and some bread. These four types integrate into my recipes so stock up.

Bananas, apples, potatoes and onions: Bananas and apples are great to eat as a snack, naturally, and you'll notice that bananas and apples are in many of my baked goods.

Tuna packets or cans: Easy-to-use pre-cooked, prepared chunks of tuna. Tuna can be easily used for salads, sandwiches or meals.

Oatmeal: Delicious to eat on its own or with chocolate chips for breakfast. I also add oatmeal here and there to various meals for fiber.

Pancake Mix: A great starting point to then add flax seed or wheat germ to.

Tortillas: Try out the Mission Low Carb ones, they are super soft and keep well.

Nuts: Almonds, cashews, walnuts, and pecans are a super nutritious food. Planters just came out with portion-sized packs of nuts, which makes for an easier way to grab and go!

Energy bars: If you're averse to energy bars you have to try my favorite: Luna Bars. The flavors will have you thinking your enjoying a treat, and the fortified, filling nutrition makes for another healthy snack.

Bags of pasta: Pasta, one of the easiest meals known to man. Always have some bags of pasta in your store. When you're short of inspiration or time, just throw some pasta into a boiling pot, and cook up a pasta sauce with extra veggies.

Vanilla whey protein powder: A nutritious supplement that's really easy to integrate into your drinks, meals or baked goods.

Box of non-fat milk powder: Mainly, it's for adding to recipes.

Low-fat evaporated milk: You get twice the protein, twice the calcium with this milk - great for cooking. Try it for home made mac-n-cheese!

Lunch-size paper plates: Use lunch-sized plates for perfectly sized adult portions. With these, you'll won't overeat, and if you clean your plate, you can still recycle!

Sweet Staples

Wheat flour and white flour
White, brown and powdered sugar
Cinnamon
Vanilla extract
Baking powder and baking soda
Can of whipped cream and tub of whipped topping.
Semi-sweet chocolate chips: Both mini and regular-sized.
Unsweetened cocoa powder

Red vines About the healthiest treat out of a plastic container, the main ingredient is wheat flour! Dipping them in chocolate is divine.

Mini marshmallows how about some cereal treats!

Nutella hazelnut chocolate spread what's it good on...anything!

Gourmet chocolate bars Eating these for dessert slows me down to really savor the unique chocolate flavor, since I paid bigger money for them.

2 cans of pie filling: I always want two, so I'm never short if I need an easy potluck dessert.

Light cereals: These are great for cereal treat recipes – who doesn't want their dessert fortified with 11 vitamins and minerals?

Solid cereals: My favorites are oat squares or chocolate mini wheats. Eat 'em dry, straight from the box as a sweet snack.

Pre-packaged 100-calorie cookie snack packs: Easy-to-open (and easy-to-eat) when I need a quick, low-maintenance sugar fix.

Popsicles and vanilla ice cream sandwiches: Good portion sized sweets.

Slow-churned ice cream: It's actually low fat—just as creamy but healthier!

White and chocolate boxed cake mixes: Great to have on hand for a super-quick baking session with kids (Jell-O cake) or for my dump cobbler cake.

"Do not be too timid and squeamish about your actions. All life is an experiment. The more experiments you make the better."

-Ralph Waldo Emerson

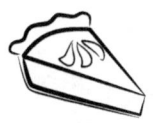

Part II: Delicious Meals

Recipe Tips

Don't be afraid to substitute, add, or delete parts of any recipe. Just as I was writing this book, it occurred to me to add a grated carrot to the breakfast cookies and pancakes. All of sudden they contained 5 food groups! Improvisation like this is really key to making healthy, inspired dishes. And this way, you'll never get bored with cooking.

There are so many healthy ingredients that you can undetectably add to meals! Even for the pickiest palate, a little touch of healthy flax seed probably will go unnoticed and perhaps enjoyed.

When trying out these recipes, don't worry if you don't have an ingredient. If you're missing flax seed, just add a tiny bit more flour to make up for it.

If changing recipes makes you uncomfortable and you start thinking worrying thoughts like, 'What if it doesn't turn out right?', then maybe altering them is the thing *TO do*! Adding or deleting components in a recipe isn't life threatening. It pushes you to think beyond a recipe card. Taking initiative like this could be a great first step towards kitchen creativity.

When I've started a recipe and I suddenly realize that I don't have all the ingredients, I'm pushed to be creative. They say necessity is the mother of invention, and when I'm in need of a missing ingredient, I'll simply get unusual!

Take one scenario: I started making my Coffee & Cream French Toast. Mid-way through mixing up my ingredients, I discovered that I didn't have milk. I wanted to complete the recipe since it's the main way my son gets eggs in his diet. So instead of rushing out to get milk, I went around the problem by substituting orange juice for milk. And, you know what? It turned out great—with a subtle hint of citrus.

All my meals are well-rounded and super-quick. They each have a 30-minute prep-and-make time. To have a little more fun, try to beat the 30 minute timeframe. What can I say, I have so much more fun when I turn everything into a game!

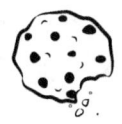

Chapter One:

Breakfast Makeovers

Great news, ladies: these recipes will help you kill two birds with one stone. The breakfast cookies and pancakes are sweet tooth-approved and they also include all five food groups! Beat that, Martha Stewart! In each recipe you'll find whole-grain-carbohydrates, egg and nut protein, dairy, fruits and even the odd vegetable. Regardless of what meal your kids will have for lunch, give them a great start with healthy meals like this. Some easy-to-integrate nutritious extras are ground flax seed (rich in omegas), whole grains (added fiber), and yogurt (filled with active cultures).

When dirtying bowls and utensils, I tend to make big batches so clean-up is less often! Eat some, refrigerate some and freeze the extra!

Breakfast Cookies

Servings: 32 (2-inch cookies). Calories: 185 per cookie.

When asked what we ate for breakfast, my kids and I get a kick out of saying we had chocolate chip cookies! If that little tickle isn't enough to make you love this treat, surely the combination of filling peanut butter and melting chocolate are enough to show you the way. Add 1/2 cup cocoa powder, and 2 tsp cinnamon for a Mexican Chocolate kick!

Time-saving tip: Freeze some dough to bake fresh cookies next week.

1. Preheat oven to 350° F.

2. Mix together:
   1 1/4 cups white flour
   1/2 cup wheat flour
   1/4 cup ground flax seed
   1/2 cup non fat powdered milk *or vanilla whey protein powder*
   2 cups oats
   1 tsp baking powder
   1 tsp salt

3. In a separate large bowl, melt and let cool one stick of butter.

(continued)

4. Add in:
> 1 stick of butter, melted
> 1 1/2 cup brown sugar
> 1 cup apple sauce *(or 1 grated apple or 1 smashed banana)*
> 1 finely grated carrot *(or zucchini) (optional)*
> 3/4 cup peanut butter
> 1 egg + 3 egg whites
> 2 tsp vanilla

5. Add dry ingredients to wet and mix.

6. Fold in:
> 1 cup semi sweet chocolate chips
> 1/2 cup raisins *(optional)*

7. Drop by large tablespoons on cookie sheet (line tray with parchment paper for easy removal and clean up).

8. Flatten dough a bit so they're the same sthickness.

9. Bake 9 min.

Chocolate Monster Protein Pancakes

Servings: 16, Calories: 100 per serving.

I care about my family's health. I want to make sure that what I'm making in the kitchen gives them what they need. With this recipe, my first goal was simply to increase protein by adding extra eggs to the box mix, since my son doesn't like to eat eggs alone. Then I just kept adding healthy ingredients. They're so chock-full of great stuff that they end up coming out like healthy little muffin tops!

Time-saving tip: This breakfast recipe is a batch large enough to split and store for another day!

Picky-palate tip: For the veggie, use the finest grater so that it's camouflaged.

1. Start with 1 fruit (mashed banana, grated apple with skin, pear, or peach)

2. Add and mix into the fruit:

   1 egg + 3 egg whites

   1 cup non fat milk

   1/2 cup vanilla yogurt

   1 tablespoons olive oil

   1 grated carrot *(or 1/2 zucchini)*

(continued)

3. Add in:

1 1/4 cup pancake mix

1/4 cup wheat flour

1/4 cup ground flax seeds

1/4 cup oats

1/4 cup cocoa powder *(for dark chocolate batter)*

1/2 cup chocolate or butterscotch chips *(or 1/4 cup of each!)*

4. Then, add 1/2 cup of our favorite cereal (optional). For bulky cereal, let the kids smash it in a plastic baggie. Or add frozen blueberries to a few.

5. Dollop thick batter onto griddle. Cook on med-low heat for a bit longer than typical pancakes since they are hearty! Serve without syrup, for less sugar and mess! If we're running late, my kids and I eat them in the car.

Coffee & Cream French Toast

Servings: 4, Calories: 375 for 2 slices with banana topping.

I made this up while pouring coffee from my French press. It smelled so delicious and rich, I just wished coffee could be in everything!

1. Mix together:

    2 eggs + 2 egg whites *(or 3/4 cup liquid eggs)*
    1/4 cup low fat milk
    1 tsp cinnamon
    2 tablespoons coffee (brewed or make instant)
    1 tablespoon sugar

2. Soak 8 pieces of bread (whole grain bread for more fiber) in mixture.

3. Place on lightly greased pan or griddle. Cook until turns golden.

4. Top these with sautéed bananas. Take 2 sliced bananas and sauté until soft in:

    1/2 cup water
    1 tablespoon butter
    1 tablespoon sugar
    1 tsp cinnamon

Chocolate Chip Oatmeal

Serving: 1 (2 packets), Calories: 500 (oatmeal with milk, nuts, flax seed and chocolate)

If your home is like mine, the plain oatmeal packets are avoided. I buy variety packs, which come with plain packets. I use up those plain oatmeal packets that no one wants by mixing them with a packet of flavored oatmeal. Who eats just one oatmeal packet anyway? (I always use two for a meal.) Mixing in milk as opposed to water, gives you added calcium. Then to spice it all up: throw in a small handful of mini-chocolate chips. Who can resist! Add some nut and seed healthy stuff and you're good to go!

1. Mix two packets of oatmeal. Go ahead and use up that plain packet, or use quick or old fashion oats in the bigger container.

2. Pour in some milk and heat up.

3. Fold in:
   tsp flax seed
   handful of chopped walnuts
   mini-handful of chocolate chips
   frozen blueberries (helps cool it quickly)

Deb's Banana-Apple Bread

Servings: 24 slices (makes 2 loaves, 12 slices per loaf), Calories: 225 per slice.

This recipe is easy enough, and is full of many healthy and sweet ingredients. My family makes this on weekends or after school. Baking it after school makes the house smell amazing while I'm working and my kids are doing homework. And what better reward to motivate completion of homework than some freshly baked banana bread!

You can cut recipe in half for only 1 loaf.

1. Preheat oven to 350° F.

2. Mix the following:
   4 ripe bananas smashed
   4 large eggs + 2 egg whites
   1/2 stick melted butter
   1/2 cup oil
   1 1/2 cup packed brown sugar
   2 tsp vanilla extract
   1 cup milk
   1 cup applesauce
   1 tsp banana extract (optional for extra banana-y taste)

(continued)

3. Mix the following in a separate bowl:
   2 1/4 cups white flour
   1 cup wheat flour
   1 cup oats
   1 tsp salt
   1 tablespoon cinnamon
   1 1/2 tsp baking powder
   1 tsp baking soda
   1/2 cup ground flax seed

4. Mix dry ingredients into the wet mixture.

5. Pour into 2 lightly oiled loaf pans.

6. Bake 45-50 minutes. Check after 40 minutes, if the top starts looking brown, place a piece of foil on the oven rack above it to stop it from burning.

Vegan Banana Bread

Servings: 8, Calories: 225 per serving.

Even without having any eggs you can make this quick bread. I can't believe what sweet, soft and pillowy bread this recipe produces!

1. Preheat oven to 350° F.

2. In medium bowl mix:
   2 cups flour *(for more fiber you can use 1 cup white and 1 cup wheat)*
   4 banana, smashed
   1/2 cup brown sugar
   1/4 cup oil
   2 tsp vanilla
   1/2 tsp baking soda
   1/2 tsp salt

3. Pour into 8 x 8 oiled or sprayed pan.

4. Bake for 35 minutes. Cool 10 minutes, or just cut immediately for faster consumption!

Lox Scramble

Servings: 1, Calories: 300 per serving.

1. Heat 1 tablespoon olive oil in saute pan or use non-stick spray.

    1 egg plus 3 egg whites (or liquid egg whites)

    1/4 non fat milk

    smoked salmon, from package, cut in pieces

    green onions or red onion diced

    capers

    1 small tomato, diced

2. Mix in bowl

3. Saute egg mixture stirring as it cooks. Top with a dollop of whipped cream cheese.

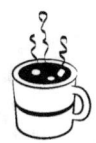

Chapter Two:

Room-Saving Meals

This sweet-lover is definitely a fan of main meals. I focus on making well-rounded meals for my family so that everyone gets the nutrients needed to concentrate on homework or work and the energy needed for after-school activities or workout sessions.

Each of these main meals feature four to five food groups. Follow the recipe I've offered and feel free to alter to your taste or wants. Finish them off with salt and pepper to taste. Get that hearty meal before moving on to a treat!

Mom's Sweet Chili

Servings: 6, Calories: 300 per serving.

This meal is very kid-friendly! Growing up this meal was a regular in our home. After missing out on my mom's delicious chili for 18 years when I was away at college and jobs, I have my mom making it for us again! We get it every time we visit. I never realized how much I loved this family crowd pleaser until after I had missed it for so long!

Bonus Recipe: Cornbread is perfect with this meal. Follow the directions on a box mix, and add one small can of creamed corn and one extra egg.

1. In 2 tablespoons of olive oil, sauté the following for 2 minutes:
   1 diced yellow onion
   6 stalks of diced celery

2. Add 1 lb. of lean ground turkey and brown for about 5 minutes.

3. Add the following:
   1 can of kidney *(or any red)* beans (don't drain)
   1 can of pinto *(or any white)* beans (don't drain)
   1 can of tomato soup
   1 can of tomato paste

(continued)

4. Add the following to your taste:
    salt
    pepper
    chili powder
    salsa
    hot sauce
    garlic powder

5. Simmer for 1 hour, take lid off to reduce liquid if needed.

6. Top with grated cheese, sour cream or black olives to serve.

Mom's Meatloaf

Servings: 4, Calories: 380 per serving.

As I kid, I grimaced at this word. 'Really?! We're having meatloaf?' It just not the most appetizing word. But it always tasted great and now I'm passing down my mom's recipe. In my house, this is kid-tested and kid-approved.

Bonus recipe: Use this to make meatballs on pasta night or meat patties on hamburger night.

Bonus recipe: Make your own bread crumbs by buttering, toasting, and then crumbling 2 pieces of bread.

1. Preheat oven to 350° F.

2. Mix the following:

    1 lb. of lean ground turkey *or ground beef*

    1 cup yellow onion, diced finely or grated

    2 carrots, grated *or one diced red pepper*

    1 zucchini, grated *or 1/2 cup chopped spinach*

    2 eggs

    1/2 cup bread crumbs

    1/2 cup grated cheese

    1 tablespoon soy sauce *or garlic salt or sea salt*

(continued)

3. Form into loaf pan.

4. Top with 1/4 cup BBQ sauce.

5. Bake for 35 minutes.

Tuna or Chicken Casserole

Servings: 8, Calories: 350 per serving.

I guess I love these all-food-groups-in-a-pan meals because I was raised on them or because they just make sense. Either way, I'm glad my kids eat and enjoy meals that don't require standing over the stove for hours (I do look forward to morphing into a higher end chef in the years to come.) Quick, easy, tasty. It's as simple as that, at least for now.

Time-saving tip: Buy packages of real pre-cooked bacon, or pre-packaged pieces of real bacon.

1. Preheat oven to 350° F.

2. Mix the following:
    1 package of egg noodles *(under cooked a tad)*
    2 cans low fat soup *(either cream of chicken or cream of mushroom)*
    1 cup milk whisked with 1 egg
    3 cans (21 oz) of tuna, drained *(or 2-3 chicken breasts poached and shredded)*

(continued)

1 package (2 cups) shredded reduced fat cheddar cheese *(mix all in or reserve half for topping)*
1 tablespoon soy sauce
2 tablespoons butter or buttery spread
4 celery stalks diced *(or 1-1/2 cups peas or frozen edamame beans)*
1/2 cup bacon pieces

3. Put mixture in casserole dish, covered in foil for 30 minutes.

4. Top with remaining cheese and 1 cup of crumbled potato chips.

5. Bake last 5 minutes uncovered.

Beef Stroganoff with a Veggie Twist

Servings: 4, Calories 550 per serving, using lean ground beef or top sirloin with fat trimmed.

Growing up this was a family favorite. I LOVE IT. I've used sherry, white or red wine and they all taste good. When I have an open bottle of something, I'll make this.

1. Boil 1 package of your favorite pasta, or cook rice or a few potatoes.

2. While pasta boils, sauté in pan:

   2 tablespoons oil or butter
   1 shallot or onion, diced, or even just onion powder, salt and pepper.
   1 lb. (2 cups) of beef (sliced top sirloin or lean ground beef for least fat, or can use any style of steak e.g: chuck roast.)

   Remove from pan, put in a bowl.

3. Use same pan to sauté:
   2 tablespoons butter
   1 container sliced mushrooms

(continued)

4. To the mushrooms, add:

   1/8 cup worcester sauce

   1/4 cup wine

   1 cup chopped spinach or zucchini

   1 can beef broth

   4 tablespoons corn starch or flour

5. Add 1 cup light sour cream and cooked meat to saute pan. Simmer for a few minutes then serve over noodles, rice or potatoes.

Thai Pork with Veggies

Servings: 8 (for a 2 lb. tenderloin) Calories: 500 per serving.

When I have a small dinner party, this really looks impressive (but it's super easy.) The sauce reduces down - in and around the meat, and it's delicious. With the coconut, lime and soy flavors it lends itself to be served with rice. And since the oven's on, might as well use it to cook some veggies too!

1. Preheat oven to Broil.

2. Make rice, or have precooked frozen rice on hand to heat up.

3. Slice a whole pork tenderloin into 1/4" slices.

4. Mix the following:
    1 cup light coconut milk
    2 tablespoons lime juice
    1 tsp sugar
    1/8 cup soy sauce

(continued)

5. Lay aluminum foil on 2 baking sheets with edges or 2 - 9x13 baking dishes. Lightly oil or spray with cooking spray. Place slices of pork in a single layer and pour mixture over it. (If both dishes don't fit side by side on top oven shelf, rotate them once or twice up to broiling shelf.)

6. Broil for 30 minutes.

7. While pork cooks, make veggies. Throw your favorite veggie, or all of the following veggies: asparagus, sliced zucchini or red peppers (quartered) on a baking sheet drizzled with olive oil and sprinkled with garlic salt. Bake for 10 minutes on the 3rd baking shelf while the pork finishes up. When taking the pork out, move veggies up to top shelf and broil for 5 minutes.

Meat & Veggie Pasta

Servings: 4, Calories 300-400 per serving (depending on meat and additions).

Sometimes I just need to do an easy dinner, and this is it! I like that I can serve it plain to my son, then add bacon, artichokes, and cheese to the pot for my daughter. After serving my daughter, I can continue adding more veggies for my final plate.

1. Boil 1 package of your favorite pasta.

2. While pasta boils, cook 1 lb. of meat on stovetop. Choose ground turkey, lean ground meat, diced chicken breasts, shrimp, scallops, whatever you have.

3. To the meat, add 1 jar of marinara sauce, or 2 cans of diced tomatoes.

4. To add some more flavor, add any or all of the following:
   1/2 bag frozen spinach
   1/4 cup real bacon pieces
   1 can artichokes
   20 sliced green olives
   handful of capers

5. Top with parmesan cheese, to serve.

Mac - n - Cheese

Servings: 4, Calories: 450 per serving (without the additions.)

Finally tired of Kraft, and having evaporated milk on hand, I came up with a great meal! Evaporated milk is the secret!

1. Boil package of pasta for 5 minutes. Drain, set aside.

2. In sauce pan mix:
   1 can Evaporated Skim Milk
   1 package (2 cups) shredded cheddar and jack cheeses
   1/4 cup flour
   2 pats butter

3. Add cooked pasta to cheesy sauce as well as bacon pieces or chicken for your meat. Add spinach, broccoli or edamame for a veggie and there's 4 food groups!

4. Other good additions are sun-dried tomatoes, italian sausage, ham, mushrooms.

Scallops or Chicken with White Beans & Bacon

Servings: 4, Calories: 254 per serving.

This is the highest maintenance dish I make, and here's the story behind it. I bought fresh scallops at Costco one day when the fresh-catch seafood case was placed front and center, catching everyone's attention. I couldn't afford the beautiful king crabs or lobsters, so I went for the palm-sized scallops. When I got home, I simply used what I had on hand to come up with this recipe! Improvising with the limited items on hand creates things you know you'll like because you stocked the basic items in the first place!

Time-saving tip: On Mondays, I poach, sauté, or bake 8 chicken breasts. I use some and store the rest in containers for easy-use later in the week.

1. Cook 2 pieces of bacon in a skillet. Remove bacon and break into pieces, set aside. (Or use packaged real bacon pieces and then 2 tablespoons oil for the next step.)

2. In the same pan, sauté 1 chopped onion.

(continued)

3. Add the following to the same pan:

    1 clove of minced garlic and sauté for 30 seconds (or garlic in a jar.)
    1 can of white beans (drained)
    1 bag (or frozen package) of spinach, cover and let wilt (about 5 minutes)

4. Preheat a separate pan over medium high heat with 1 tablespoon each olive oil and butter.

5. Add 1 lb. of scallops (blotted with a paper towel) or chicken tenders.

6. Sear until brown about 2-3 min per side. Be careful not to crowd the pan or they will steam, not brown.

7. Serve scallops or chicken over veggie mixture and sprinkle with bacon.

Tortilla Soup

Servings: 6, Calories: 300 per serving.

This is a best friend's recipe. I love it because she'll make it for me when I go over for dinner. Everyone needs a good role model and a friend like her. So in her home, during dinners like this, I try to embody my *eat-like-a-child* eating style. Slowing down to relish all the moments of the meal makes it even better.

Isn't it funny how a normal soup recipe can be a such a great meal, when you know it's made with love?

1. In a stew pot, combine:
    1 can (32 oz) chicken broth
    1/2 bag baby carrots (diced)
    1 large unpeeled potato (diced)

2. Bring to gentle boil.

3. Sprinkle garlic powder on 2 chicken breasts and sauté with a tablespoon oil n pan, set aside, dice when cooled.

(continued)

4. In separate pan, sauté in 2 tsp oil for 2 minutes the following:

   1/2 yellow onion (chopped)
   2 stalks of celery (diced)

5. Add 1/2 small can of red enchilada sauce to the veggies.

6. Add everything to the stew pot.

7. Simmer for 5 minutes.

8. Top with tortilla chips, cheese, cilantro, sour cream to serve.

Enchiladas

Servings: 8, Calories: 450 per serving.

My four girlfriends and I used to make dinner for each other. It was great while our kids were young. Knowing I'd only have to make one meal per week, it was a big load off my shoulders. But of course that one meal was prepared for 5 families! So I had to be prepared. At 6pm on my designated weekday, I'd drive my family to my friend's homes to deliver our meal. Such a great bonding experience that really helped us all! Enchiladas was one of the tastiest meals that was easy to multiply into giant portions.

1. Preheat oven to 300° F.

2. In a big bowl, combine:

    4 chicken breasts, cooked shredded
    1 rectangle of cream cheese
    1/2 package (or can) of frozen corn
    1 can mild diced green chilies
    1/2 cup cheddar cheese
    1 avocado, smashed (optional, or use on top.)

3. Place mixture in tortillas and roll into big enchiladas.

4. Put them all in a baking dish, pour mild green enchilada sauce over it.

5. Top with 1/2 cup cheddar cheese and bake 30 minutes covered in foil, 5-10 minutes uncovered.

Mexican Lasagna

Servings: 4, Calories: 400 per serving.

Okay, you're probably thinking that I really love my tortillas. Yes, you'll discover that meals with a touch of Mexican cuisine are real big time savers, and just like Taco Bell, come from the same 5-6 ingredients.

With some ground meat or turkey, a taco flavor packet, and tortillas, you already half-way to a having dinner prepared! This lasagna-type dish is super quick and easy. You get the same meal as self-assembly burritos or tacos, minus the mess of numerous bowls and tabletop spills.

1. Preheat oven to 350° F.

2. Oil the bottom of a baking dish.

3. Start with a tortilla on the bottom, layering the following:
   tortilla
   seasoned lean ground meat
   your favorite canned beans
   diced green or white onions
   salsa
   shredded cheese

(continued)

4. Repeat the layers two more times.

5. Bake 30 minutes.

6. Top with cilantro and black olives to serve.

Baked Ziti with Spinach & Tomatoes
Servings: 8, Calories: 325 per serving.

My college roommate taught me this easy recipe! It's got all the components of the food pyramid. I make this for many block parties or potlucks. It's huge hit with kids and adults alike. Try it out and see that dinner-time can be hassle-free! Make it and freeze half for another week.

1. Preheat oven to 375° F.

2. Cook in large saucepan, medium high heat:

    12 oz chicken sausage, casing removed
    1 medium onion, diced
    3 cloves garlic, diced

3. Sauté for 10 minutes, drain fat.

4. Stir in:

    1 can (28 oz) of diced tomatoes
    1/2 cup store bought pesto sauce

5. Simmer until thicker.

(continued)

6. Boil water and add 10 oz ziti pasta, undercook.

7. Drain and add:

   6 oz package of spinach (frozen works too)
   8 oz mozzarella cheese, shredded
   1/3 cup Parmesan cheese, grated
   tomato mixture
   meat mixture

8. Transfer to baking dish. Sprinkle with 2/3 cup
   Parmesan cheese.

9. Bake 30 minutes.

Bean & Cheese Potato
Servings: 4, Calories: 350 per serving.

I have to admit, I just really like beans and cheese and want to put them on everything. But you hardly had to guess! A potato serves as a good variation to a tortilla.

1. Pierce 4 medium potatoes with a fork a few times and microwave for 3-5 minutes. Be sure to check every 2 minutes since microwaves vary.

2. Top with:
   black beans
   cooked chicken
   salsa
   diced green chilies
   low-fat sour cream or cottage cheese
   some shredded cheese

Twice-baked Potato
Servings: 4, Calories: 300 per serving.

Another best friend taught me this recipe. It's super easy, the only thing you have to remember is to start it one hour before you actually want to eat, which is why I don't make it too often. I seem to wait until the last minute to figure out dinner, so I'm often strapped for

(continued)

prep time. So, I invite this best friend over as often as possible, to enjoy making this together while our kids play. Without the bacon, this meal is great for the growing trend of "Meatless Mondays."

1. Preheat oven to 375° F.

2. Pierce 2 large Russet potatoes with fork, rub lightly with olive oil and wrap in foil to bake for 45 minutes.

3. Cool for 10 minutes in refrigerator.

4. Cut in half the long way.

5. Scoop out insides and mix with:
    butter
    sour cream
    grated cheese
    cooked broccoli
    diced green onions
    real bacon pieces

6. Bake again for 10 minutes, this time at 325° F.

BBT Slaw

Servings: 4, Calories: 125 per serving.

BBT stands for **b**acon, **b**roccoli, and **t**omato! And I'll say broccoli twice, because it tastes so nice! In all seriousness, I like coleslaw, but when I saw broccoli slaw (shredded broccoli stems in a bag), I just about jumped with excitement. I love firsts, and broccoli slaw is a unique twist on a yummy classic.

I came up with this recipe when I agreed to bring a side salad to a function. I looked at the recipe on the bag that called for cranberries, and I didn't have any on hand. But I did have real bacon pieces. With mayo and diced tomatoes it tasted like a BLT!

On many occasions, I've eaten this entire salad for lunch. But hey, it's a bunch of veggies with a healthy dose of meat and nut protein! You'll find this seriously irresistible. Consider yourself warned, ladies.

1. Mix the following:

   1/4 cup real bacon pieces
   1 bag broccoli slaw (or bagged lettuce)
   1 cup diced tomatoes
   1/4 cup light mayo
   1/8 cup rice vinegar
   2 tablespoons sugar
   1/4 cup sunflower seeds (or sliced almonds)

2. Serve in a medium-size bowl or pack up for lunch.

Chicken, Rice & Veggie Casserole
Servings: 6, Calories: 310 per serving.

I make this when I hit the oh-my-gosh-I'm-really-hungry moment. It's a quick dish that's extremely filling. If there ever was an easy dish with the highest fill-factor, this has to be it.   With the chicken breasts that I precooked on Monday, and with the frozen cooked rice, you'll cut corners even faster.

Bonus recipe: To vary this dish, add any veggie like spinach, zucchini, edamame.

1. Preheat oven to 350° F.

2. Combine the following:

    2 cups shredded Monterey Jack cheese (equals one bag sold at grocery stores)
    2 cups cooked rice (frozen bag of it comes in handy)
    1 1/2 cups cooked, chopped chicken breast meat
    1 can low or non-fat evaporated milk
    1/2 cup grated onion
    2 large eggs, lightly beaten
    1/2 cup chopped spinach (frozen, drained) or sliced zucchini
    1/2 cup grated carrots (can buy packaged this way)

(continued)

    2 tablespoons butter, melted
    1 handful of chopped cilantro (optional)
    1 tablespoon diced jalapeños (optional)

3. Stir well.

4. Lightly grease 2-quart casserole dish, and transfer mixture into dish.

5. Bake for 30 minutes.

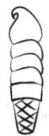

Chapter Three:

Simple Meaty Meals

These easy meals don't require pot or casserole dish. I simply make fish, chicken or pork using the stove, oven, or even microwave for a ever quicker cook times. Serve with sides of your favorite veggie and carb, or throw it on top of a big salad! I'm not skilled at the outdoor grill, but if you are, it seems like a fabulous tool!

Easy Fish

Servings: 4, Calories 200 per serving.

1. Some mild fish choices are cod, tilapia, snapper, or orange roughy.

2. Thoroughly season 4 fish filets with Creole seasoning, or Panko bread crumbs mixed with garlic salt.

3. In a large frying pan, melt 4 tablespoons of butter (or heat 1/8 cup oil).

4. Pan-fry each side on high about 3 minutes until crisp.

5. Remove fish and sauté sliced zucchini or asparagus in the same pan.

Can make rice simultaneously in rice cooker or heat up the frozen cooked rice that you've purchased.

Simple Shredded Pork

Servings: 4, Calories: 225 per serving.

1. In a big pot, over med-high heat, sear a pork tenderloin in 2 tablespoons of olive oil.

2. Sear 3 minutes per side, or until easy to lift up and flip.

3. Add big jar of mild green salsa or big can of green enchilada sauce.

4. Simmer covered for 1-3 hours on low or in a crock pot.

5. Use 2 forks to pull it apart into shredded pork.

Tastes great when served with tortillas (big surprise), lettuce, tomato, avocado. Add 180 calories per serving for all these ingredients.

Easy Chicken 1

Servings: 4, Calories 200 per serving.

1. Coat 4 skinless chicken breasts with Dijon mustard, soy sauce, lime and garlic mixture. Alternatively BBQ sauce or Italian dressing work too. Or try Dijon and BBQ sauce mixed together!

2. Cover and microwave for 4 minutes, then flip over for another 4, power level 8. My mom bakes it covered for 40 minutes at 250° F, depending on thickness. Baking for a longer time at a lower temperature makes really tender chicken breasts.

3. For a side: microwave some veggies (broccoli, zucchini, edamame, asparagus, baby carrots tossed with 1 pat of butter or olive oil, 1/8 cup water and salt) covered for 4 minutes.

Easy Chicken 2

Servings: 4, Calories 275 per serving.

1. Preheat oven to 450° F.

2. Coat chicken with mustard.

3. Then press it into 1/2 cup of Panko bread crumbs mixed with 1/2 cup parmesan cheese, salt and pepper.

4. Place on foil lined baking sheet and bake 15-20 minutes.

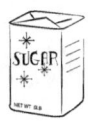

Part III: The Sweet Stuff

A Love Note to Desserts

Every person I know has at least one family member who's known for great dessert recipes. Since we've all been raised with someone creating delicious treats at home, we associate the warm feelings of comfort, family-time, and pleasure with home-baked goodies. Can it be possible for human beings to simply detach from all this goodness and cut out sugar? I would argue that it's just about impossible.

I have memories of making sticky buns with pecans, brown sugar, and butter on Christmas morning with my grandma. This is what it's all about—desserts mean love. Everyone who makes desserts loves the process as well as the fact that family and friends cherish it. There is no way to stop the love when desserts are on the menu.

There have been many times when my daughter and I started a recipe without looking in the refrigerator first, and ended up having to create a cake with no eggs. Some might call this disaster, but any challenge, presents an opportunity for me to show my kids and myself that we can be creative, resourceful and above all optimistic. We can take a difficult situation, have some fun in finding a solution, and enjoy the outcome just as much as we would have without encountering the problem in the first place.

In the case of the egg-lacking cake, my daughter and I had a ball discovering alternative ingredients. We eventually settled on applesauce and 1/4 of a packet of gelatin. We had a ball inventing something new out of our mistake.

By taking difficulties in stride and making the most out of every situation, you'll find that life is greatly improved both inside the kitchen and beyond.

When I make desserts, whether by following recipes or improvising, I create family memories and truly enjoy the quality of my family's life.

Chapter Four:

Super-Quick Daily Desserts

Those who are crunched for time might think there's no time in this world to create a delicious dessert for your family to enjoy. But even the most time-starved will enjoy these simple and fast fixes. They are a breeze to make—and eat, if I do say so myself.

Desserts can be a hassle-free delicious treat that's enjoyed at the end of a long day or after a hearty meal. In order to create home-baked treats you don't need buckets of time. Try a few of these, and you'll see that getting your sugar kick is easier than ever, and can be enjoyed warm, straight out of the oven. Plastic-wrapped treats don't stand a fighting chance!

Without further ado, here are a few of my super-quick daily desserts.

Oven S'mores

Servings: 8, Calories: 145 per serving, 180 with sautéed bananas

If I went camping every week, I might get my fill of S' mores. But since I don't, I had to think of a substitute! These can be made individually in the microwave heated for 20 seconds (a big marshmallow triples in size as it heats - fun to watch with kids) or in the oven for a larger batch.

Time-saving tip: Use mini marshmallows-- they'll melt faster than big ones!

1. Preheat oven to 250° F.

2. Line a cookie tray with foil for easy clean up.

3. Lay out 16 square graham crackers.

4. Top each with 8 crackers with semi sweet chocolate chips. Top the other 8 crackers with mini marshmallows.

(continued)

5. Bake for 5 minutes in the oven. Use toaster oven for mini batch.

6. Put chocolate crackers and marshmallow crackers together for 8 S'mores sandwiches!

7. Optional: Sauté a banana in pat of butter and enjoy on top of open-faced S'mores!

Dump Cobbler

Servings: 12, Calories: 308 per serving

Straight from college I jumped right into the workforce. Without any free time to hone my baking skills, I was thrown into the deep end when it came time to bring a dessert to a social event.

To my first dinner party, I brought this dump cobbler unbaked. I was over-worked and out of time. Something needed to be pulled together quick for my hosts. I threw in what I could and wished for the best.

Baking this cobbler at the hosts' home ended up being the highlight of the evening! The whole house filled with its sweet smell. This became one of my stand-by desserts. Cherries are my favorite filling, and the cobbler tastes best with ice cream.

1. Preheat oven to 350° F.

2. Dump 2 cans pie filling in 9x12 dish.

3. Dump 1 box white or yellow cake mix on top.

4. Drizzle 1 stick melted butter over the cake mix.

5. Bake for 30 minutes uncovered.

Chocolate-dipped Goodies

Calories: 140 per 1/8 cup of chocolate chips (then add calories for item dipped)

Be imaginative and take anything in your pantry really, to discover a new treat by dipping it into melted chocolate. Some of my favorites are red vines, pretzels, ginger snaps, strawberries, and coconut macaroons. You'll be surprised, but, potato chips and Fritos are another great dipping treat!

I have a fondue pot, but it's stored high up in my pantry and so it's inconvenient to bring down. Not to mention, cleaning a fondue pot and all it's parts is not the most forgiving task in the world. To bypass the fondue madness and simply get down to enjoying some chocolate-dipping, try this simple trick.

1. Melt 1 cup of semi sweet chocolate chips in microwave for 2 minutes.

2. Stop to stir every 20-30 seconds until smooth.

3. Dip your choice of snack halfway into the chocolate.

4. Lay on waxed paper to cool.

5. Place in refrigerator for faster results!

*"Some dreams of fortunes,
others dream of cookies."*

-Note from a fortune cookie

Chapter Five: Easy Cereal Treats

These cereal treats actually fit under the **Super-Quick Daily Desserts** chapter (page 25), but they are so amazing that they deserve a chapter all to themselves.

Cereal treats lighten up the mood and bring smiles to everyone's faces. No event is too big or small - corporate meetings, PTA meetings, barbecues, plane-ride snacks, birthday parties, bake sales, holiday block parties—you name it. This easy-to-serve and quick-to-make treat is perfect for any occasion.

I even brought them to a friend's bachelorette party in Las Vegas. When my 30-year old friends saw me walking in with a tray of crispy rice treats, they laughed. But guess who devoured them all later that night? Everyone! People will smile (or chuckle) when they see a plate of cereal treats. They'll think it's only a kid's dessert. But once they taste that crispy, crunchy sweetness, fun memories will flood back and instantly they'll be smiling because they're so happy you brought them.

You'd be surprised, but all cereals work well. My favorite mix is 4 cups clustery, flakey, or granola cereal and 5 cups rice cereal (total of 9 cups cereal). Don't be shy: use any kind of cereal you can get you your hands on. The results will always be super tasty.

A serving of marshmallows is comparable to fruit's sugar content, gram for gram. Rice cereals are fortified with essential vitamins and minerals with little sugar. And chocolate chips add antioxidants to your cereal treats! Of course, I'm just joking here. No one's advocating the superior health benefits of marshmallows over that of fruit. But, hey, if you're going to eat dessert, it's great to know that the sugar-content is relatively low and that there are some nutrients in these little goodies!

Grab your biggest stew pot, because these ingredients really add up to a lot of volume.

Deb's Benchmark Recipe for Cereal Treats

Servings: 24, Calories: 105 per serving.

1. Melt 3 tablespoons butter with a <u>large bag</u> (16 oz) of mini marshmallows.

2. Remove from heat.

3. Add 9 cups rice cereal *(or try mixing any two.)*

4. Spread into 9x13 dish or large cutting board - it's a big batch!

Special Cocoa Krispies Treats

Servings: 24, Calories: 252 per serving.

1. Melt 4 tablespoons butter and 24 oz of mini marshmallows in big non-stick pot.

2. Add whole boxes of both Cocoa Krispies and Special K Chocolaty Delight. Mix in evenly.

3. Spread out and cool on large cookie sheet or cutting board. Oh my gosh, are they good!

Family Favorite Cereal Treats

Servings: 24, Calories: 120 per serving.

My favorite: 5 cups Cocoa Krispies and 4 cups Recess Peanut Butter Balls.

My daughter's favorite: 5 cups Rice Krispies and 4 cups Cinnamon Toast Crunch

My son's favorite: 5 cups Rice Krispies and 4 cups Crispix.

Cereal Mud Patties

Servings: 20, Calories: 112 per serving.

1. Melt 1 package semi-sweet chocolate chips.

2. Mix in a box of cereal. Try a fiber cereal—you're treats will look like muddy haystacks. Use any other kind of cereal if fiber cereal doesn't appeal.

3. Blob onto wax paper and cool in refrigerator for faster results!

4. To get more to go around, cut blobs into quarters or halves.

Cereal Chow

Servings: 20, Calories: 225 per serving.

This light, crunchy treat is filled with a flavorful chocolate-peanut butter kick!

1. Melt:

    1 bag semi-sweet chocolate chips

    3/4 cup peanut butter

    1 stick of butter

2. Add 9 cups Rice Chex, Crispix, Oat Squares or other sturdy cereal.

3. Toss mixture in plastic bag with 2 cup powdered sugar to coat all the pieces.

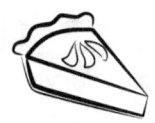

Chapter Six:

Desserts Worth Working For

These amazing baked goodies might be a touch more time consuming than the previous super-quick treats. But getting your family into the kitchen to create some memories is definitely worth the extra time. With sultry doses of sugar, chocolate and butter, they are nothing but captivating. Some things just aren't meant to be healthy. I'm sure with one whiff of these baking in your oven, you'll definitely agree.

"Good bakers never lack friends." -Anonymous

Papa's Chocolate Bread Pudding
Servings: 8, Calories: 320 per serving.

My ex-husband's dad is a great cook and baker. Now I get to call him my *father-out-law* and I'm his *daughter-out-law*. I've always enjoyed working with him in the kitchen. We went through a phase of making and eating bread pudding. Through the process we uncovered some great recipes and came out with some very full bellies! Here's his take on our most favorite bread pudding recipe.

1. Preheat oven to 325° F.

2. Bring to simmer in medium saucepan the following:
    1 cup whipping cream
    1/2 cup sugar
    1/2 cup whole milk

3. Remove from heat, add 1 cup chocolate chips

(continued)

4. In a separate bowl whisk 1 large egg and 1 tsp vanilla.

5. Gradually whisk in the chocolate mixture.

6. Add 4 oz of French bread cubes. Throw in the remaining 1/4 of chocolate chips and toss everything together.

7. Transfer to shallow baking dish. Sprinkle with sugar and bake 50 minutes. The sugar topping will become crunchy after baking—what a delight!

Whipped Cream

Servings: 16, Calories: 105 per serving.

A restaurateur friend of mine told that adding Irish Cream liqueur is the key to great whipped cream. Whenever I do, it's a crowd pleaser!

1. Place metal beater part and bowl in freezer to chill for 15 minutes.

2. Beat 2 cups of cream slowly in cold bowl, gradually increasing speed.

3. Add the following:

   1 tablespoon sugar and
   1/2 tsp vanilla (optional)
   1 tablespoon Irish Cream (optional, then no vanilla needed)

4. Serve immediately or store in airtight container in fridge.

Mom's Turtle Cake

Servings: 16, Calories: 285 per serving.

Go, mom! This cake is gooey and super yummy! It's a crowd-pleaser, so it's a great potluck dessert.

1. Preheat oven to 350° F.

2. Prepare 1 box chocolate cake mix.

3. Pour 1/2 into 9" x 13" pan and bake 15 minutes.

4. Melt 1 bag Kraft caramels and 1/2 cup of low-fat evaporated milk over low heat.

5. Pour over hot cake. Sprinkle 1 cup chocolate chips and 1 cup chopped nuts on top of caramel. Pour remaining batter on top.

6. Bake for 18 more minutes. Careful, because this cake will be soft until the caramel is set.

Maple Pumpkin Cheesecake

Servings: 12, Calories: 392 per serving.

This is a *Better Homes and Gardens* recipe that I came across when looking for a Halloween party dessert. This is seriously an amazing cake, well worth the careful techniques and extra thought. I rarely use my Cuisinart machine or spring form pans. But for this cake, I'm always happy to pull them out and put them to good use.

The crowd will sigh when you drizzle caramel syrup on top when serving. You can add candied pecans and whipped cream to add some more flair.

1. Preheat oven to 325° F.

2. For the crust, mix the following:
   1 1/2 cups (20 squares) graham cracker crumbs or ginger snaps
   1/3 cup sugar
   5 tablespoons (stick) melted butter

3. Press onto bottom of 9" x 13" glass dish or 9" spring form pan.

4. Bake 8 minutes.

5. After completing the crust, readjust oven to 300° F.

(continued)

6. For the filling, beat the following:
     24 oz (3 packages) cream cheese
     1 can sweetened condensed milk
     2 cans pumpkin puree
     1 tablespoon whipping cream
     1/4 cup maple syrup
     1/2 tsp all spice
     1 tsp cinnamon

7. Beat 3 eggs into mixture one by one.

8. Pour mixture into pie crust.

9. Bake 1 hour and 15 minutes. Cool for 15 minutes on stovetop or wire rack, so air circulates under it.

10. Run knife around cake and open the spring form pan to cool further for 1 hour.

11. Put cake in refrigerator for 4 hours before serving.

Really Great Chocolate Chip Cookies

Servings: 18 cookies, Calories: 160 per cookie.

This is a *Cook's Illustrated* recipe. One of my best friends introduced me to this supreme recipe. Together we've made countless batches. As I write this, she's planning to move shortly. So now when I bake this recipe without her, I'll smile with happiness, remembering all the wonderful memories and kitchen talks. And I'll probably even cry from missing her and wanting to bake this with her again. Thank you, *Cook's Illustrated,* for offering such a great recipe which has fostered so many unforgettable moments!

1. Preheat oven to 325° F.

2. Mix in a medium bowl:

    2 1/8 cups all purpose flour
    1/2 tsp salt
    1/2 tsp baking soda

3. In a large bowl, melt 12 tablespoons (1 1/2 sticks) unsalted butter and cool.

(continued)

4. To the butter, mix the following:

    1 cup brown sugar

    1/2 cup white sugar

    1 large egg + 1 yolk

    2 tsp vanilla extract

5. Add dry mixture to wet mixture and mix well.

6. Stir in 1 1/2 cups semi sweet chocolate chips.

7. Drop large spoonfuls on a cookie sheet.

8. Bake 12-15 minutes until golden brown around the edges and still puffy in the center.

9. Cool on baking sheet.

Double Chocolate Chip Cookies

Servings: 12 cookies, Calories: 125 per cookie.

I'm always looking for variations on a good thing. I added cocoa to a great cookie recipe and it was a hit with friends at our holiday cookie party.

1. Preheat oven to 375° F.

2. In large bowl, beat the following:

    1/2 cup brown sugar
    1/2 stick butter until fluffy
    1/2 tsp. vanilla
    1 egg

3. Add the following:

    3 tablespoons unsweetened cocoa
    1 cup flour
    1/2 tsp baking soda
    1/8 tsp salt

4. Stir in 1/2 cup semi-sweet chocolate chips.

5. Drop spoonfuls on a cookie sheet.

6. Bake 8 minutes.

7. Cool on cookie sheet.

Oatmeal Chocolate Chip Sugar Cookies

Servings: 24, Calories: 210 per serving.

My creative son says "Mom, can we make a chocolate chip *sugar cookie* and have it be oatmeal too?" You can tell we like all cookies, so why not combine them!

1. Preheat oven to 375° F.

2. In large bowl, mix:

   1 1/2 stick butter, melted
   1/4 cup sugar
   2 tsp. vanilla
   1 egg + 1 yolk
   1 box white or yellow cake mix
   3/4 cup flour

3. Fold in 1 cup of chocolate chips.

4. Drop large spoonfuls on a cookie sheet.

5. Bake 8-10 minutes.

6. Cool on cookie sheet.

Moist, Double Chocolate-Vanilla Cake

Servings: 16, Calories: 330 per serving.

This is a delicious chocolate cake with chocolate chips (or half white chocolate chips if you have 'em!) Make it in a bundt pan and dust with powdered sugar or top with a vanilla glaze for an elegant look. (Or bake in a 9 x 13 pan and finish with whipped toping and possibly crunched up chocolate cookies for a more playful feel.)

1. Preheat oven to 350° F.

2. In large bowl, beat the following:

   4 eggs
   1/2 cup non fat milk
   1 cup vanilla yogurt
   1/2 cup oil
   1 package chocolate cake mix
   1 small box instant chocolate pudding mix
   1/4 cup flax seed and 1 cup chopped spinach for a health kick; it's a topic of conversation at parties!

3. Fold in 1 1/2 cups chocolate chips (or 3/4 cup chocolate chips and 3/4 cup white chocolate chips.)

4. Generously spray bundt pan with vegetable oil spray, pour in mix and bake 45 minutes.

5. Invert pan onto serving plate.

*For an awesome **Vanilla Apple Spice Cake** use a Spice Cake box mix with vanilla pudding and add 2 diced or grated apples (I also grated a carrot and dumped that in too.) Or for a delicious **Butterscotch Bake Cake**, use a Yellow Cake box mix, butterscotch pudding and butterscotch chips instead.*

Vanilla Sugar Glaze
Servings: 16, Calories: 50 per serving.

In small bowl mix:
- 1 cup powdered sugar
- 1/4 cup milk
- 1 tsp. vanilla extract

Then drizzle it over the cooled cake!

Variations of Glazes:

- 1 cup powdered sugar
- 1/4 cup any flavored liqueur

For example: Irish cream, coffee liqueur, raspberry schnapps or orange liqueur (Triple sec) would make the glaze have a hint of that flavor.

- 1 cup powdered sugar
- 1/4 cup milk
- 1 tsp any cooking extract.

For example: Cherry, banana or peppermint extracts would give the glaze a hint of that flavor!

Beach Crumble

Servings: 16, Calories: 200 per serving.

This wonder is named for its blue**be**rry and pe**ach** components. Ingenuity shapes new successes, so don't let a lack of ingredients halt your dessert making! I thought to make a berry crumble, but only had 6 cups of frozen berries—not enough for my recipe. Then I saw my ripe, juicy peaches, so I combined the 2 fruits to make up the 9 cups of fruit needed!

1. Preheat oven to 375° F.

2. For the filling mix all ingredients:

   4 cups blueberries (frozen okay)
   5 cups peaches, diced, skin removed (frozen okay)
   1 cup sugar
   4 tablespoons corn starch
   1 tsp cinnamon

3. Place in 9 x 13 baking dish.

(continued)

4. For the crumble topping, mix the following:

    6 tablespoons butter, cold, cut into pieces
    1 cup oats
    1 cup flour
    1 cup brown sugar
    1 tsp cinnamon

5. Use a knife (or even fingers) to crumble the butter into the dry ingredients.

6. Pour on top of filling mixture in the baking dish.

7. Bake for 50 minutes.

Caramel Corn

Servings: 8, Calories: 175 per serving.

It's best if I'm full before making this. It's so utterly scrumptious I would eat it all if hungry! A fun variation for movie nights.

1. Preheat oven to 325° F.

2. Pop 1 bag of microwave popcorn (I like lightly buttered popcorn).

3. Remove un-popped kernels.

4. Put popcorn into a big roasting pan, and keep warm in preheated oven.

5. For caramel mixture, in a medium saucepan, combine:

> 3/4 cup brown sugar
> 6 tablespoons butter
> 3 tablespoons light corn syrup

6. Cook and stir until boiling. Let boil at low rate without stirring for 5 more minutes.

(continued)

7. Remove saucepan from heat.

8. Stir into sugar mixture:

   1/4 tsp baking soda
   1/4 tsp vanilla

9. Pour this caramel mixture over popcorn, stirring gently to coat. Bake for 10 minutes.

10. Stir mixture. Bake 5 more minutes.

11. Spread caramel corn on buttered foil to cool. Store for 1 week in airtight container.

Jell-o Cake

Servings: 12, Calories: 350 per serving.

2 steps of fun, right here! After making and baking the cake, pour liquid Jell-o over it. When cut pieces are served, you can see the colorful Jell-o drizzle marks throughout the cake and it tastes like whatever flavor. (2 flavors is even better - One blue and one red make for a great 4th of July cake!)

1. Prepare white cake (follow directions, add milk instead of water for more protein and calcium.) Bake it in a 9x12 baking dish, cool it.

2. Poke the finished cake with a fork A LOT, all over it, at least 100 times.

3. Make 1 box of Jell-o (with 1/2 cup less water) and pour liquid jello over white cake, slowly.

4. Refrigerate for 2 hours.

5. Top with cool whip and serve!

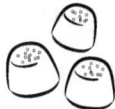

Chapter Seven:

Desserts with a Dash of Healthy

Here are some lighter options to mix it up a bit. These are easy, tasty recipes that, you could even say, dance the line of healthy.

No-fat Chocolate Cake

Servings: 8, Calories: 210 per serving.

This one's for my mom, who loves to omit fat from recipes.

1. Preheat oven to 350° F.

2. In medium bowl mix:

    1 cup flour (for more fiber you can use 3/4 white and 1/4 wheat)
    1/2 cup unsweetened cocoa
    1 tsp baking soda

3. In a separate large bowl, beat:

    6 large egg whites
    1 1/4 cups brown sugar
    1 cup non-fat vanilla yogurt
    1 tsp vanilla

4. Stir in flour mixture.

5. Pour into 8 x 8 oiled or sprayed pan.

6. Bake for 35 minutes. Cool 15 minutes, then top with powdered sugar or whipped cream from a can!

Coconut Macaroons

Servings: 18, Calories: 105 per serving.

This recipe is basically from the Baker's Coconut bag. I'm a macaroon enthusiast. I've tried making more complicated recipes, but this recipe with my added egg white and extra flour is totally satisfying! Egg whites have loads of protein, which help balance the sugar intake as well as all the essential amino acids your body loves.

1. Preheat oven to 325° F.

2. Mix:
    a bag of coconut shavings
    2/3 cup sugar
    8 tablespoons flour
    1/4 tsp salt

3. Stir in 5 egg whites and 1/2 tsp of almond extract.

4. Drop by tablespoons onto parchment-lined cookie sheet.

5. Bake for 20 minutes. Remove immediately and cool on wire rack.

Doctored-up Brownies

Servings: 16, Calories: 245 per serving.

Take an average box of brownies and doctor them up to create a real treat. I've tried three different brownie recipes from scratch. But nothing beats this doctored-up version of my Ghirardelli box mix.

The discovery process was a near scientific feat! So excited to uncover the secret of brownie making, I made four batches of brownies one right after the other. Brownies overflowed from my kitchen as I arranged four taste-testing platters for my neighbors and kids. In the end, the doctored-up brownie won.

This doctored recipe is a shining example of a healthy sugar kick.

1. Follow box directions to create brownies.

2. Use olive oil in lieu of vegetable oil if you want. No worries, you can't taste it in finished product.

3. Use milk instead of water for more calcium and added protein.

(continued)

4. Add an extra egg yolk.

5. And the main twist of imagination: Add 1 cup of finely grated zucchini or 1 cup of spinach chopped (fresh or frozen).

6. Bake in oven for time and temperature specified on box.

Soda-baked Apples

Servings: 4, Calories: 90 per serving.

Baking these apples make the house smell amazing.

1. Preheat oven to 350° F.

2. Peel, core and cut 4 apples into halves.

3. Place apples in baking dish.

4. Pour in 1 can cola or cream soda.

5. Sprinkle with cinnamon.

6. Cover with foil and bake for 45 minutes.

Grilled Dirty Bananas

Calories: 150 for each dirty banana.

When camping for a week, I got creative with our S'mores ingredients.

1. Wrap whole bananas in foil and put on grill over campfire.

2. Turn occasionally and after 20 minutes, unwrap.

3. Slice open lengthwise, leaving skin on.

4. Crumble chocolate and graham crackers on top on warm banana.

5. Scoop out with spoon. Fun to eat and super delicious.

Tri-Ingredient Chocolate Soufflé

Serving: 1, Calories: 175 per serving.

In my house, our love of dessert is almost a religious commitment. That's why I jokingly call my kitchen the church of glucose. With a sweet tooth craving and limited ingredients on hand at the end of the week, I churned out this beauty for a sugar fix, some great protein and anti-oxidant benefits. It's good, easy, stuff.

1. Mix the following in a big coffee mug:

> 2 tablespoons unsweetened cocoa powder
>
> 2 tablespoons powdered sugar
>
> 1 egg + 1 egg white

2. Microwave the mug for one minute.

3. Try not to smile too big as it rises up and tilts like the leaning Tower of Pisa!

4. Add chocolate chips (better) or top with whipped cream (best). It's an easy single-serving dessert with some protein!

Grilled Chocolate Sandwich

Servings: 1, Calories: 320 without nuts (375 with nuts).

The perfect lunch! Think I'm joking, now, do you? Try this and you'll be tempted to eat this at any time of the day.

Healthy knowledge bite: For 12 years, I was a vegetarian. During that time I learned that by combining a nut and a whole grain, a nut and a legume (beans and peas), or a whole grain and a legume you can get a complete protein! Drink some soymilk with this whole grain sandwich and you'll get a complete protein!

1. Preheat griddle or pan.

2. Lightly butter 2 pieces of whole grain bread.

3. Put semi-sweet chocolate chips and nuts (optional) inside.

4. Grill each side until crispy like you would a grilled cheese sandwich!

Banana's Foster

Servings: 2, Calories: 250 per serving.

When vacationing in Mexico, this delight was available at any restaurant. I loved it so much that I took a mental note of what the waiters were doing at my table. Here's what I came up with.

1. Preheat sauté pan.

2. Melt:
    1 tablespoons butter
    1/8 cup brown sugar
    1/2 tsp cinnamon

3. Add 2 bananas cut in slices to the pan, as well as 1/8 cup banana liqueur or water. Optional: add 1/8 cup dark rum, if you're feeling like a flavorful kick.
Can omit all alcohol and simply add ¼ cup water to sauté bananas with.

4. Sauté for a few minutes. And pour over Vanilla Ice Cream!

Nutella & Banana Crepe

Servings: 6, Calories: 225 per serving.

I have a fond memory of eating lunch out with my childhood best friend at a crepe restaurant. We got a savory crepe and a sweet crepe. We shared the two between us and enjoyed every single minute. Living in a small town without a crepe restaurant, it became imperative that I learn how to make this in order to honor that wonderful memory.

1. Sauté 2 bananas as in Banana's Foster, no liqueur or rum needed.

2. Make a thin pancake batter with pancake mix or by mixing the following:
   2 tablespoons salted butter
   2 eggs
   1 cup milk
   1 cup flour

3. Pour 1/4 cup of batter onto heated saucepan.

4. Flip carefully.

5. Once done, place on plate, spread with Nutella and sauteed bananas. Fold over sides of crepe like an open ended burrito.

6. Don't forget to top it with whipped cream.

Lemony Bars

Servings: 16, Calories 105 per serving.

I was deprived of lemon-flavored things growing up since it wasn't my dad's favorite flavor. With this somewhat-healthy Lemony Bar, I'd like to think that I'm making up for lost time!

Time-saving tip: Don't have the materials on hand? Despair not! Substitute 3/4 cup of flour for the flour-flax combination, can use all white flour instead of wheat flour.

1. Preheat oven to 350° F.

2. For the healthified crust, mix the following in a small bowl:

    1/4 cup wheat flour

    1/4 cup white flour

    1/4 cup ground flax seed

    3 tablespoons sugar

    4 tablespoons cold butter, cut in chunks

3. Keep cutting butter smaller and smaller until it's a crumbly mixture, or use fingertips to press flour into butter.

4. Press lightly into 8" x 8" pan coated with oil.

(continued)

5. Bake 15 minutes. For the time-starved and perhaps just plain starved, you could just stop here and eat this healthy-ish shortbread-like cookie crust.

6. For those who want to press on, create the filling by beating 3 eggs until frothy.

7. Add the following:
    2/3 cup sugar
    3 tablespoons flour
    3 tablespoons lemon juice

8. Beat on medium speed for three minutes.

9. Pour into crust-lined pan.

10. Bake for 25 minutes.

11. Cool for an hour on wire rack or gas stove top, so air gets under it, or place in fridge to chill quicker.

12. Sift powdered sugar on top to serve.

~

Share your thoughts or feedback! Tell me the things you love. Feel free to send along any health and fitness tips or family recipes, and I'll post them in my blog!

~

Connect with Debbie Online:

Facebook: Functionably Happy

Twitter: Debbie Markham

Blog and Website:www.functionablyhappy.com

email: debbiemarkham@functionablyhappy.com